THE
MAN DIET

CHAD HOWSE WITH
STEPHEN ANTON PH.D

Legal Disclaimer

Warning: All the information presented in The Man Diet is for educational and resource purposes only. It is not a substitute for, or an addition to, any advice given to you by your physician or health care provider.

Consult your physician before making any changes to your lifestyle, diet, or exercise habits. You are solely responsible for the way information in The Man Diet is perceived and utilized, and doing so it at your own risk.

In no way will Chad Howse, Dare Mighty Things Publishing, or any persons associated with The Man Diet be held responsible for any injuries or problems that may occur due to the use of this book or the advice within it.

Personal Disclaimer

I am not a doctor, and although Stephen Anton is, does not mean that our advice should replace your doctors. Any advice given in the book, if you choose to follow it, should be discussed between you and your doctor.

Results Disclaimer

Required Legal Disclaimer: Due to recent laws from the FTC, it is required that all companies identify what a "typical" result it. The flat out truth is that a typical result is nothing, no gains, no health improvements, not boosts in testosterone because a "typical" person doesn't act, they don't go to the gym, they don't sleep 8 hours a night, they don't get their body fat under 14%, and so on. The testimonials I share on various pages on my web sites are not typical, they're pictures of action takers who exercised and ate well. If you want those same results, work hard and implement what we cover in this book.

Copyright Notice
Published by: Dare Mighty Things Publishing

CONTENTS

Introduction. 1

Chapter 1 - The Emasculation 3

Chapter 2 - The Man Hormone 11

Chapter 3 - How to Become the Wolverine 21

Chapter 4 - TESTOSTERONE. 25

Chapter 5 - Testosterone Routine. 29

Chapter 6 - Testosterone and Life. 33

Chapter 7 - What is Testosterone? 37

Chapter 8 - Things You Can Do to Boost Your Testosterone Levels Naturally 41

Chapter 9 - The Do's 43

Chapter 10 - Don't. 63

Chapter 11 - The Daily Testosterone Routine. 73

Chapter 12 - Keeping Optimal Testosterone Levels During the Day 91

Chapter 13 - The Testosterone Evening 99

Chapter 14 - The Man Diet 103

Chapter 15 - How Your Current Diet is Ruining Your Masculinity. 107

Chapter 16 - A Guide to Eating Like a Man. 111

Chapter 17 - What to Do. What to Avoid. How to Eat Like a Man. 131

Chapter 18 - How Much Should You Eat? 139

Chapter 19 - Testosterone-Boosting Foods 147

Chapter 20 - Your Simplified Schedule. 157

Conclusion. 161

About the Authors.. 163

Other books to read: 167

Resources: 169

Citations 171

Part II Citations 183

INTRODUCTION

"Over-sentimentality, over-softness, in fact washiness and mushiness are the great dangers of this age and of this people. Unless we keep the barbarian virtues, gaining the civilized ones will be of little avail."

– Theodore Roosevelt

THIS BOOK HAS been almost a decade in the making. As you'll read in the coming chapters, it started with a chance meeting and an introduction into the world of testosterone. From there I've spent as much time sifting through myth and nonsense as I have spent showing other men what works.

While the book focuses on diet, and it will show you how to eat optimally, and in a way that you can sustainably eat for the remainder of your life while enjoying what you eat, it's also a book I wrote to help both myself and other men figure out how to live optimally. The goal is to regain those 'barbarian virtues' that Theodore Roosevelt talks about, but are being driven away and replaced with the softer virtues that anyone and everyone can possess, but benefit few.

We'll talk about manliness and masculinity, however, as it pertains to testosterone. And while the Man Diet is heavy on nutrition and how you should eat, increasing testosterone is as much a battle of the mind and lifestyle as it is of food.

In later chapters, you'll discover how making money and winning a competition sends your testosterone levels through the roof, and how losing and stress sends them plummeting. While I'm going to show you how to eat like a man, turning your back on the feminine diet books that litter bookstores all across this continent, I'd be doing you a disservice if I didn't also talk about how lifestyle and mind-set affect testosterone as well.

So we'll cover it all.

You'll learn how to eat, how your government's food pyramid is upside down, how your environment can be killing your testosterone levels and how these hormone levels regulate how you take risks in life, but also how healthy you are.

If you want to eat a healthier diet, this book is for you.

If you want to have better sex with your lady, you've found the right reading material.

If you want to win, to kick ass and take names, again, you have found the right book.

This book will permit you to eat like a man, live like a man, and act like the man. You'll learn the truth about testosterone, diet, and how living with those necessary barbarian virtues as your base, will allow you to be better, stronger, and more dependable for those who look up to you and need you to lead them.

Let's get after it.

Chad Howse

Chapter 1
The Emasculation

Masculinity is not something given to you,
but something you gain. And you gain it
by winning small battles with honor.

~ *Norman Mailer*

YOU WEREN'T MADE to be a sedentary being living a monotonous life. You weren't placed in the time and space in which you were born merely to exist. You aren't a lap dog. You aren't a coward. You aren't created to be fat or weak or continuously afraid of doing what your soul begs you to do.

Men are bred to fight. We're born to conquer, to venture into the unknown, to explore. One-half of our species can get pregnant; the other half can't. The mere fact that men cannot bear children makes it necessary that they defend them and those who can. It forced the masculine half of our species to be more aggressive, to be physically stronger, to be more prone to taking risks of the physical nature, each of which is spurred and driven by our most powerful hormone, testosterone.

The difference between them and us - our ancestors, the hunters, and gatherers, the warriors and conquerors and explorers - is drastic.

We once hunted beasts with spears and arrows and our bare hands. Now what do we do? Sleep? Watch others live? Buy things to impress people we don't even like? Exist in a community where our only form of competition is determining who has the best lawn or the fanciest car in the driveway?

Too often what we do with our time is beneath what our capacity, our potential should dictate we do, and why we do it is also driven by motivations that are beneath us, our species, and what men once were and in some places, some small pockets of society, still are.

There's a feeling that with the decline of masculine values like self-reliance, self-responsibility, and grit, we're seeing a drop in who men are on a social level. We're producing fewer fathers who act as fathers should. We're creating fewer men who do what they can with what they have, while also producing more complainers, criers, dependents, and whiners.

While we may be producing more pussies who are afraid to defend themselves and fight for what's right and even identify what's right, that isn't you. While there very well may be a decline in masculinity, something I agree with, there is a decline in men, and it's been scientifically proven.

Our society needs men just like they need women, and they need men to be men and women to be women.

From a hormonal standpoint, this isn't happening like it once was. Men are quickly being feminized. If you take the two sexes, forget about the fact that men can't get pregnant and women can, making their roles in a tribe dramatically different, and look exclusively at what makes us different chemically and hormonally, we have a very different hormonal makeup.

Women are on one side of a spectrum, and men on the other. The further men get from their end, the closer they get to that feminine side of the equation. The result of this decline in men from a hormonal standpoint is seen in the side-effects of low testosterone on a grand scale.

- *Increases in depression amongst men, and suicide.*
- *Increases in heart disease and prostate cancer.*
- *A fatter population with less muscle mass.*

A decline in testosterone, which is exactly what researchers out of Massachusetts found, is a decline in the quality of human that you or I can be. And while the solutions we'll cover in this book may be relatively simple to apply, the causes for this decline are quite complicated. (*The Journal of Clinical Endocrinology & Metabolism*, Volume 92, Issue 1, 1 January 2007, Pages 196–202, https://doi.org/10.1210/jc.2006-1375)

The most in-depth study on testosterone in current male populations is the one listed above, that you can read more about here:

https://academic.oup.com/jcem/article/92/1/196/2598434.

From that study:

*The estimated cross-sectional decline in TT is −0.4% per year of age, with a corresponding 95% confidence interval (CI) of (−0.6%, −0.2%). The longitudinal within-subject decline is approximately −1.6% per year (CI: −1.8%, −1.4%). **The age-matched time trend is −1.2% per year (CI: −1.4%, −1.0%).***

…the typical blood sample taken from a 65-yr-old man in 2003 exhibited lower TT concentrations than a sample taken from a different 65-yr-old subject in 1988 (the latter subject having been born approximately 15 yr earlier than the former).

*…These findings indicate that the past 20 yr have seen substantial **age-independent** decreases in male serum T concentrations.*

In short, male testosterone levels are decreasing dramatically and it doesn't matter what your age is, you're likely being affected. It's as if our men are becoming less masculine, and not just socially, but biologically and physically. Your grandfather's testosterone levels were way higher than your own. This study is frightening, yet few seem to give a rat's ass. We don't see a rush to study this decline, one that has many adverse effects on the male population (we'll get into most of them), like we do the rush to study other ailments - though this decline seems to be the cause of many of the other things we see so much funding for.

My goal is to reverse this downward trend one guy at a time.

The more guys that read this book, the greater the impact. For now, let's focus on you. How can you create the thriving testosterone levels that were once the norm? How can you improve your male hormones so they can help you live the life you want to lead?

As a guy in my mid-twenties (now in my thirties), testosterone wasn't on my mind at all. I was supposed to be in the prime of my physical life, so I wasn't aware of the signs of low testosterone. I thought how I was feeling was normal. I also didn't know how powerful optimal testosterone levels could be, that is until I had a bloody accident...

The Epiphany

So here I stand...

...half way up a volcano in Maui. The lush greenery is like nothing I've ever seen – which is saying a lot coming from Vancouver. It's cold and its wet. Goosebumps cover my skin like spots on a cheetah but the smile on my face has never been wider.

Due to some beautiful ingenuity and a fair amount of free time, the owner of the property – the one on the side of the mountain that I'm standing on – has dug a trench down the slope that winds like a snake slithering along the sand moving from side to side from tail to head, ending at a small pool at its base.

He's lined the two and a half foot trench with a slippery rubber-like material creating one of the steepest and longest water slides I've ever seen. Brilliant.

I'm about to go on my 4th or 5th run, each time going faster and faster, and I make the decision to hold nothing back, to push the limits of this thing and hope I don't fly off either side, or worse, skid along the lava rock that lines the edge of the pool at the bottom of the slide.

I'm there with a group of 10 or so people. All of whom have done numerous runs down the side of this mountain. Some face first. Others are on their back. Others were going in groups. Each is trying to push the limits while finding the balance between fun and stupidity. I get it into my head that fun is stupidity and the more stupidity in your actions the more fun they will be.

I determine that it's my butt that's slowing me down. My shorts are dragging me behind a wee bit so on this run I decide to have only my heels and my upper back touch the slide, after, of course, a short sprint at the top of the slide to gain enough speed pre-launch. Which I do successfully, and I'm off!

I'm *immediately* struck by the reality that I'm going way too fast, but what can I do but try and go faster?

Turn one almost sees me launched off the side but by the skin of my left butt cheek I hold on and cruise down at top speed. Finally, on the last dip down to the home stretch I gain way too much speed and am propelled off the left bank of the final turn and slide stomach and face first into the well-placed lava rock surrounding the pool.

For what seems like minutes I slide across the lava rock before I'm dumped into the pool. It stings a little, but it doesn't seem so bad. Getting out of the pool, blood starts pooling around my chest and arms making my forefront look like a peeled raspberry.

It looked like I was skinned. Bleeding profusely I walked back up to the top off the hill, everyone else half in shock that this happened, half laughing because of the sight of me launching from the final turn of the slide, and partially concerned about the blood starting to drip from my chest, stomach, and knees.

Thankfully, only a few months earlier, I'd begun an experiment...

CHAPTER 2
THE MAN HORMONE

*"You have to be a man before you
can be a gentleman."*

–John Wayne (McLintock!)

AT THE TIME, I was young. Maybe I still am depending on your perspective. I was supposed to be in my physical prime, but that's not how I felt.

I was in my early twenties, and I'd recently begun feeling lethargic and even a bit depressed. I'd gained fat for the first time in my life and after having competed in boxing for a few years; I was, for the first time in my life, without a sport. Gone was the competition I loved so dearly, and in its stead, the good ol' 9-5.

I was lifting weights to look better for the first time in my life, and it just didn't feel right. As such, I was eating to gain lean muscle, following the guidelines of various experts on what that entailed, eating high amounts of carbs and lean proteins and very little fat.

You could say I was in a funk, but it felt like more than a funk. It felt like something systematic and treatable was bringing me down, and I was too damn young to lose my 'mojo' – both literally and in life. My life was feeling like it was average, boring, and mundane. It wasn't because it was mundane, but because I wasn't chasing things like I was previously. I wasn't setting massive goals, and I didn't have big wins. I wasn't taking risks…

…Even something as simple as that waterslide…

That's a sign of high testosterone, trying to push yourself more than everyone else, even take unnecessary risks. As you'll read, testosterone levels decline when men have families. They think this happens because of that risky behavior, the jumping off of cliffs, going out into the wilderness alone, exploring, and so on and so forth, doesn't benefit husbands, who need to be alive and well to earn a living for their families, so they become safer and more sedated.

This isn't the story for history's *greatest men*, though. I just finished reading, *Farther Than Any Man*, the book about Captain James Cook, one of the best adventurers and explorers this planet has known. That's a man. He's a guy who needed to explore, and that need wasn't quelled when he got a family, it was only increased.

Our hormones may want to tell us to calm down, to be more safe and average and normal, but that's not what's best for us. We can spur on our optimal testosterone levels both by how we act and how we eat. For a while there I was slipping into this mediocre, monotonous existence that has always scared the hell out of me. I wasn't going hiking, going to the boxing gym, doing things that may be a little dangerous, I wasn't as assertive or aggressive, I was bland, and I was starting more and more to live a dull life.

You may think this is just life. But it isn't. It never is. There's always a choice to become the man that will spark a better life. There's always the choice to take risks, to embark on adventures, to set your sights higher. I was getting weaker, more tired, and less excited about life.

Now, some reading may see this as depression. Well, depression is increased when you have low testosterone.

This went on for a while.

Even though I'd built that size I wanted, I started an online business to Help guys do the same, there was still this feeling that things weren't right.

What I didn't know then, was that each of these symptoms are signs of low testosterone. Heck, I didn't even know that testosterone was a good thing! I thought it was a rage-inducing hormone that we can only increase by synthetic means, like shots or creams.

My 'ah-ha moment' came in the form of an introduction.

I was in New York for a quick trip and I lined up meetings with guys who were making big moves, both in my industry and other areas of business and life (at least I was trying to *force improvement*, to force growth and to see how winners are living - I'll give myself that). One such new friend invited me up to his apartment for breakfast. On the menu: 6 eggs each and three slices of bacon per person (everything I'd been told is horrible for you).

Today we're a bit more knowledgeable about dietary fats and their effects on our hormones, but back then I had no clue and asked why the hell he was feeding me so much damn fat – even though I was *dying* for some bacon.

His answer was earth-shattering…

…Because fats increase testosterone.

My immediate response was, *testosterone?*

That hormone I'd been told came from drugs my entire life, he explained, was the most important hormone for men to have optimized.

He explained some of the signs of low testosterone…

He mentioned that I should be waking up every day with a hard-on, that if I'm carrying more than 14% fat then it's likely that my estrogen levels were too high, or that if I wasn't getting at least 7 hours of quality sleep every night, that it was very likely that my cortisol levels were too high, and that one of the ways we measure testosterone is in relation to cortisol. If your cortisol levels are too high, your testosterone levels automatically can't be high enough. He talked about my lack of dietary fats, and that if I'm not consuming enough fat that I'm not feeding my testosterone levels. We talked and talked and holy hell was I interested.

This was years ago. We know a lot more about testosterone now, but this was my introduction to the hormone that makes men, men, this was exciting shit! I began to see a reason for my malaise. The worst is when you're feeling like crap, but you have no cause, no source that you can focus on, change, and create a cure. You may feel like crap, but at least when you understand why, there's some hope, even better, some enemy you can defeat.

As soon as I got home, I went to the doctor and got my levels tested. The results weren't catastrophic, but they also weren't optimal. There was work that I could do.

No guy wants to hear that they have less than optimal testosterone levels. In our society, we measure ourselves many different ways. If you're with your pals and it slips that you have low T, Your good buddies are going to relentlessly bust your balls. You don't want to give them that material. And you don't want to feel like you're a diminished version of who you once were. You have to keep in mind that there's a decline across men of all ages, too. It sucks. But your old man had higher T levels at your age than you do, and your grandfather had higher T levels than your old man. You're in a time of low testosterone, but this isn't a bad thing, necessarily.

As I soon discovered, when you understand the causes, you can create a solution, and your competition on this planet and in this society has never been weaker.

Not to jump from topic to topic but this has to be covered…

It's never been easier to be successful.

Think about both the market and your competition. We live in the vainest, most materialistic society of all time. We're a consumer society, and the market has never been more hungry for good products, nor willing to fork over the dough. So the demand is there, but there are also more people, so wouldn't that mean that the competition is even stiffer? NO! We're also the most entitled society us humans have ever produced.

People don't want to work. They don't want to persist.

If they're willing to work, they want results right now. Take it from me; I'm in a business that does not see a lot of persistence. In the online world there are a few instant success stories, but far more stories of people who quit. The guys who do the big things merely put the effort in for a long enough time. Your competition is entitled. They're lazy. They're a bunch of participation-trophy receiving pussies. Just by being willing to work, you're going to have a massive leg up. The same logic applies to testosterone, if you only use what I show you in the Man Diet, you're going to do what other guys are not only *not willing to do, but don't have a clue that they should be doing it.*

Back to my quest to create optimal testosterone levels...

The first book I picked up was Tim Ferris' *the Four-Hour Body*, in which he has a chapter on testosterone, using himself as a guinea pig to try to increase his testosterone levels naturally, primarily by increasing his dietary fat consumption. That book led to different studies, many of which we'll cover in this book, and a completely different outlook on how to optimize the male body.

The key word there is male.

Men and women are different. This book focused only on the former because that's where the most significant "gap" in nutrition can be found.

When I was doing my research on testosterone, I quickly found out that there's little in the way of nutrition books specifically for men. Go to your local bookstore and head to the health section. You'll find a slew of books geared toward helping women lose fat. Open them up, and you'll see meals dominated by salads and quinoa and chicken, utterly devoid of the dietary fats that produce testosterone (more on this in a sec). They're also bland and boring. When your lady tries to get you on a diet, not only is it not tasty, it's not meant for you on a hormonal level.

What I also found was that the government's food pyramid is completely upside down. They've made certain foods illegal, foods we'd thrive on if they weren't regulated (take raw milk, it's better for us than pasteurized milk, and yet it's illegal). I also found that what I've been told is Healthy from day one, isn't necessarily so.

Much of what I was eating, the containers I was using for my food and my water bottles, my shampoos and deodorants, even how I dealt with stress was all lowering my testosterone levels which was having a horrendous impact on my body, both physically and mentally.

Here's the scary part...

This decline in testosterone, a hormone that helps fight depression, disease, and cancer in men, isn't relegated to yours truly. As previously mentioned, we're seeing a decline of up to 1.3% annually, independent of age!

That kind of decline is *insane*. At that rate, we'll be walking genderless drones in a few generations.

Other studies have found that young men as young as 20 years of age who experience impotence or "can't get it up," suffer from low T as well. The decline that occurs at the age of 30 years, one widely thought to be the result purely of age, is now believed to be due to a change in lifestyle more than anything. As we age, we move less.

It indeed seems that masculinity is on a decline from a

social standpoint as self-reliance, stoic hard work, and personal responsibility appear to be relics of the past amongst the increasingly dependent majority. Though we will touch on how to become a better man, and even how to be better at being a man, our primary focus will be to fix this physical decline in masculinity that's starting with our hormones.

There is a *literal* and hormonal fall of man in that men of today aren't as manly as they once were if masculinity is defined as it is by a man's degree of testosterone flowing freely in his body. It's affecting our physical health, but also our mental health as men kill themselves at rates far higher than those of women (as a caveat, women attempt suicide at almost twice the rate of men, so maybe this suicide epidemic that men are facing has less to do with depression and more to do with the fact that we're more efficient at the act of suicide. Maybe the increases in depression in men don't need to be solved with more talking about the depression, but instead, more focus on finding a purpose that was once blatantly clear, find a job, find a lady, build a family, feed the family. With options, with ease, comes the ability to think about more than just your survival. But we can't discount this decline in testosterone and its effect as well. As we're fatter, lazier, and weaker, as we consume less wild game filled with its powerful omega 3's, our suicide rates increase. In Stephen Ilardi's, *The Depression Cure*, there were zero cases of depression found in hunter-gatherer societies worldwide. Hunter-Gatherer tribes live in a manner that's much more in line with our DNA and genetics. They also eat more meat, consume more omega-3's, and carry less body fat. They're also in a community, not an online community, but a literal community.)

Back to testosterone...

This depletion of your dominant sex hormone is happening all around you, but with the right knowledge in your back pocket, it's controllable.

This book was written to combat this 'emasculation' and reverse this decline in male testosterone levels - or at least *your* testosterone levels.

- *I'll show you how to naturally increase your testosterone levels through both diet and lifestyle changes that you can implement today.*

- *I'll cut through the incredible amount of myth surrounding natural - and unnatural - testosterone enhancement, and deliver you the truth, regardless of opinion.*

- *I'll simplify everything, so you can not only follow a 'diet' for the remainder of your life, enjoying the foods you depend on for energy and satisfaction, but create an optimal body composition while you're at it.*

This is the Man Diet. It's time that our society stopped being so bloody pussified, and we unleashed our men to be men. Let's start by eating like one.

CHAPTER 3
HOW TO BECOME THE WOLVERINE

"Because there is very little honor left in American life, there is a certain built-in tendency to destroy masculinity in American men."

–Norman Mailer

WE'RE BACK ON that mountain, blood dripping from my chest, stomach, and knees. I lie down fully expecting this wonderful vacation to come to an end. I'm a mess. The pain isn't too severe. Then someone gets a bottle of rubbing alcohol and pours it all over my stomach - okay that was a tad painful.

I thought the next few days would be spent on my back, being immobile, but they weren't, not at all.

I'd been 'eating like a man' for a few months now. Consuming more fats in the morning and at night as well as consuming a testosterone shake I'll tell you about a bit later in the book. I dropped my body fat, started supplementing with ZMA before bed, as well as maintaining a sleep schedule (sleep is one of the most critical factors in boosting your testosterone levels). I was lean, strong, energetic, and those hard-ons were there every morning once again.

Now, one of testosterone's primary jobs is to repair tissue.

That's why steroids work. They help you repair tissue so you can train 2x or even 3x as much as an average man while recovering entirely after each session. Testosterone also helps repair skin, which, of course, is a form of tissue. So with blood dripping from my body, the healing process began before my eyes.

After day 1 I was already scabbing. By day 3 I'd almost completely healed, with only a bit of light scarring. I began to notice my newly optimized testosterone levels at work in other areas as well.

For one, I woke up with a boner every damn day – which is a sign of healthy testosterone levels. Second, I noticed more attention from the ladies. Researchers have found that optimal testosterone levels result in the release of powerful endorphins that attract the opposite sex.

I'd read about both, the tissue repair and the improved sexual function that coincides with an endorphin release, but it sounded a bit fantastical. Here I was, turning heads (which is a rarity for myself), and waking up with morning wood which was something I *never did* when I was in that lethargic state before I discovered that my testosterone levels – or lack thereof – were a primary culprit.

Hence, I was healing like the Wolverine.

If you've ever read comics or seen the X-Men movies, you'll know that Wolverine's central power is his incredible ability to heal. Testosterone is, essentially, 'the Wolverine hormone' if you think about it.

It helps you repair faster, recover more quickly, all so you can damage your body and then build it back up - which is the process of building muscle and burning fat.

What follows is a look at what testosterone is and how we produce it in our bodies. To know how to increase your levels it helps to understand how it's made. We won't get too technical, but reading the next few chapters will open your eyes to the lies of both the nutrition and health industry and our government with it's insanely distorted look at diet as well as some of our doctors who don't take the time to understand how important testosterone is for men and opt to merely prescribe testosterone injections that increase their bottom line but utterly ruin our ability to produce the hormone naturally.

So get ready to get a little mad at the lies we've been told since we were wee lads, but ecstatic at the light at the end of the tunnel and the simple and easy ways you can begin to naturally increase your testosterone levels once and for all!

Chapter 4
TESTOSTERONE

*It's not the years in your life that
count. It's the life in your years.*

~ Abraham Lincoln

ANATOMY AND PSYCHOLOGY aside, men are men because of
one potent hormone: Testosterone.

We once had this hormone in spades, not merely because
of our diet (though this is a huge factor), but because of our
lifestyle, how we lived, and how frequently we moved. As
we've evolved technologically, we've *devolved* physically. As
what we eat is what we buy instead of what we hunt, and as
we've become much more sedentary, our testosterone levels
and our overall health has plummeted. This lifestyle is primarily the norm in the Western world. It's a lifestyle that has
led to a consistent, persistent decline in the average testosterone levels of men over the past few decades.

This is scary. **Men are biologically becoming
less manly.**

As I mentioned briefly, testosterone, this wonderful hormone that makes a man a man, is on the decline in men across the world. Where it was once thought to merely be a problem for men over 40, guys in their twenties are now experiencing the phenomenon that is "low T."

There are a number of causes of this dramatic decline in manhood. Many of them are around you right now without you even knowing about it. They're put on your produce, in your plastics, in your water, even in your milk and meat acting as a Trojan Horse, feeding you testosterone's enemies – cortisol and estrogen – without you even knowing it.

Our lifestyles are an attack on our most important hormone. We sit, we get fat, we live in a way that we're not genetically programmed to live.

In writing about depression in his book, *The Depression Cure*, Stephen Ildari notes that:

> *"There's a profound mismatch between the genes we carry, the bodies and brains that they are building, and the world that we find ourselves in. We were never designed for the sedentary, indoor, socially isolated, fast-food-laden, sleep-deprived frenzied pace of modern life."*

When studying the hunter-gatherer tribes that still exist in the world today, he found almost no cases of depression. When asked if they exercise, they found the concept odd. As communities, we hunted and foraged for hours per day, Typically for around 4-6 hours. Exercise was life, not a thing we did to ensure we don't get fat and die.

Genetically we, humans, namely men, are designed and evolved and genetically programmed over thousands of years to be continually moving, hunting, even competing and battling. The life we've created for ourselves that's wrought with ease and devoid of physical hardship not only leads us to be fat and weak, but it goes against our genetics, and it's incredibly destructive to our hormones.

Our diets are killing our ability to produce testosterone by making us fatter – body fat is incredibly estrogenic – but also by not feeding us the nutrients required to maintain healthy testosterone levels.

Stress, a construct of the mind and not always something that deserves the response we give it, cripples our ability to hold higher testosterone levels. Our lives have never been more comfortable in human history, yet we've never been more depressed or stressed.

Our testosterone levels are being attacked from every corner, be it our lifestyle, our diet, even the tap water we drink or the bottles we pour that water into. The vast majority of our deodorants, toothpaste, and shampoos contain chemical estrogens that artificially lower our testosterone levels.

As you can see, this book cannot and will not merely be about diet, although simple changes in your diet will do wonders for your testosterone levels. It is and has to be about more, about lifestyle changes, environmental adjustments, even mental switches we can use to reduce the stress that raises our cortisol levels – one of testosterone's mortal enemies.

This book is also not for those content as they are now. All of us, myself included in this maybe even more-so than you are mediocre in comparison to where we can be and who we can be. This book is for those of you who want more, who want excellence, who want to go beyond even where you're currently aiming. And we're starting from the ground up, from the inside out, with the hormone that makes you a man and that can potentially make you far better at being a man.

With all of that said, with the decline and the seemingly systematic destruction of the male sex hormone, there is light.

There's a lot of light.

I went from the low end of production to the high end with only simple changes to my diet and my lifestyle. It's not hard, but it does require discipline and effort. But you're a man, since when was discipline and effort a deterrent?

CHAPTER 5
TESTOSTERONE ROUTINE

"A man does what he must - in spite of personal consequences, in spite of obstacles and dangers and pressures - and that is the basis of all human morality."

~ Winston Churchill

TESTOSTERONE'S A BIG, imposing word.

It's connected to our manhood, our sense of self, and to be notified that our testosterone levels are even less than optimal, let alone downright low, is, at the very least, disheartening.

Every man's idea of himself, who he is and who he can be, is connected to his virility.

We're warriors, leaders, providers, protectors, and procreators.

Our testosterone levels are *who we are.*

To have them degraded is to have us degraded. No man wants to walk around as a shell of the man he was – or the man he thought he was.

That, however, is our reality.

The odds are that you're producing less than optimal testosterone levels. You may even have LOW testosterone levels. And just as the word, testosterone, is imposing, so is the prospect of figuring out how to once again – or for the first time – create high, thriving testosterone levels, naturally.

You, of course, can go the testosterone replacement therapy route (TRT). Which, and most guys in the natural testosterone production space won't admit this, isn't a bad option, especially if it's your only option (maybe you have a glandular problem, and your body just isn't producing it like it once was).

The problem with TRT is that it takes the place of your body's normal processes.

So when you're on TRT, you stop producing testosterone naturally, sometimes all together.

They're also expensive as shite, and **by no means are they the only way to go about it.**

Here's the thing, your body's natural form of the hormone is more potent than the synthetic form. So if you can produce testosterone all on your own, you're going to perform more efficiently, you're going to be healthier, you're going to have more energy, a higher sex drive, and you're not going to be faced with the prospect of having to take your shots all the time to feel this way.

The downside to natural testosterone production is that it's often posed as a complicated process by people who 'know better than the rest of us and sell their complicated solutions for a premium.'

It isn't.

That's what I've found out over the past decade, a decade focused primarily on figuring out how to naturally boost *my* testosterone levels, using myself as a guinea pig, testing the claims and the studies (so many studies are incredibly flawed), and providing my readers with the truth, the real information, the things they can do that will actually move the needle in their battle to produce higher testosterone levels.

There lies a massive barrier between you and your optimal testosterone levels, gimmicks. Most sources on testosterone optimization will focus on tricks. They'll talk about a root or a supplement that will be your 'cure-all' resource for improving your testosterone levels. It's all nonsense. We're going to focus on the things that will make the biggest impact, not the minor, mediocre changes that won't move the needle.

Even my own supplement company, Average to Alpha Supplements, focuses on filling the gaps we have in our nutrition that will help us lower estrogen, cortisol, and boost testosterone. Take Barbarian, for example, the Manhood Multi. It isn't a 'testosterone booster' because they don't exist. It's a good multivitamin that has things like zinc, selenium, and vitamin C, all minerals and vitamins that help with testosterone production. So don't worry about gimmicks. Don't think that a pill or a powder will help. You have to get the big things - like your weight, sleep quality, and diet - under control first before you even think about supplementation.

The actual means by which you can increase your T levels are simple; they're just not commonly known. They also make total sense. All you have to know is a little bit about testosterone, and you're halfway there.

Before we begin breaking down the routine and the diet that you're going to follow (one filled with A LOT of freedom), let's once again go over the 'why.'

When you know why you're doing what you're doing, when you understand the reason for the objective, you're far more likely to stick to the plan.

CHAPTER 6
TESTOSTERONE AND LIFE

'You don't choose your family. They are
God's gift to you, as you are to them.'

~ Desmond Tutu

MY NONNA IS a great lady. She's now in her mid-nineties which puts her in her twenties during the Second World War in Italy. My mom is also a great lady.

During that Second World War, my Nonna was in northern Italy taking care of her new family. My mom was just born as the war was coming to a close. Germans were clearing houses in my Nonna's tiny town in Italy.

When a group of soldiers got to my Nonna's house, they barged in, took a look around, but, like any new mother of any species, my Nonna didn't just sit there and let them trash her home or rough her up or endanger her young daughter, my mom. Instead, she grabbed a pot and started whacking them on the head to get them to leave.

Thank GOD a senior officer was within earshot and

heard the commotion because as my Nonna did her best to defend her home and protect her young daughter while her husband was likely in Siberia in the midst of the massacre that saw only 4,000 of 30,000 Italian soldiers return from the campaign (the things that man saw and lived through and endured, chronicled in Eugenio Corti's, *Few Returned*, prove that no matter how dark, no matter the horror or pain or tragedy we face, we can always move forward).

As she stood her ground and defended her family with a metal pan, one young soldier grabbed his gun, pulled it back an was about to clobber my dear Nonna in the head, maybe killing her on the spot, when the senior officer barged in, scolded the younger soldier for what he was about to do, and kicked the lot of them out of the house, leaving both my beautiful Nonna and my Mom in tact, healthy, and shaken from the event.

Seventy years later I'm in Canada, as are my Mom and my Nonna. I have a lifetime of lessons and gifts and guidance from both of those great women, but I was seconds away from having that taken away from me.

So what's my point?

The point is that no matter who we are, where we live, what family we're born into, we have someone who's directly or indirectly sacrificed something to give us life, opportunity, the ability to live how and in whichever manner we want.

We have soldiers we'll never know nor hear about, who laid down their lives to give us a chance at freedom. Throughout our history, as humans, we've had constant threats facing this notion that each person is an individual and able to live how they want, yet we waste this continually.

Daily we give into desires that pull us away from the men we can become and the lives we can lead.

We choose laziness over hard work, sloth over discipline, and dependency over self-reliance.

This cannot be who we are nor how we live.

I'm guessing that, for the most part, this isn't who we are. We fall into traps here and there. We're confined by limited beliefs and ways of thinking. We set goals not worthy of our talents or imagination.

We're muzzled by a society that wants to tame men, to sedate them, to make them passive and weak, and then they wonder where their protectors and defenders are.

Here you are reading about testosterone. You're actively seeking out ways to make your life better. You're actively seeking self-improvement.

You're aware of the sacrifice. You understand the notion that life is a gift and to live it in any other way than your absolute best, to have anything less than sheer ambition and audacity in how you carry yourself daily is an absolute SIN, let alone a bloody waste.

And while testosterone is but a hormone, it can serve as the foundation for a much better, healthier, more energetic and sexually active life.

You may want to boost your testosterone levels so you can have stronger and better erections. You may be seeking out this knowledge so you can burn fat easier, or build better muscle, or ward off things like depression.

You may have a *single goal*, which is great because it brought you here.

But what you're going to get is simple: POWER.

Testosterone, in the male body, is power. It acts as a reward system for winners, for guys wanting to get after it, to kick ass and take names and live a longer, healthier, better life.

The routine that follows may seem like a pure health thing, but it goes beyond that.

If you want to be at your best. If you're going to be the best man you can be (and I correctly assume that's in part why you're here), **then getting your testosterone levels to the point where they're no longer dying, but thriving, is a necessary step.**

Let's get after it!

CHAPTER 7
WHAT IS TESTOSTERONE?

"He understood well enough how a man with
a choice between pride and responsibility
will almost always choose pride—if
responsibility robs him of his manhood."

~ Stephen King

WE NEED TO know the basics, of course, and why we're doing what we're doing, but testosterone production isn't that complicated. You don't need a degree to understand how it's produced and therefore how to create more of it.

You do, however, need to understand the process.

Testosterone is a 19-carbon steroid hormone made from cholesterol.

The vast majority of your testosterone comes from your testes (important, 95%, so keep your balls cool and healthy – more on this later).

So, how is it produced?

The simple version:

1. It begins, interestingly enough, in the brain, when our hypothalamus detects that our body needs more testosterone it secrets a hormone called gonadotropin-releasing hormone. This hormone then shuttles its way to the pituitary gland at the back of the brain.

2. When the pituitary detects gonadotropin-releasing hormone, it starts producing follicle-stimulating hormone (FSH) and luteinizing hormone (LH). FSH and LH head down to our testicles via our bloodstream.

3. FSH and LH then tell our testicles to do two very magical things (this is all pretty insane and magical come to think about it). First, FSH begins sperm production, and LH stimulates the Leydig cells in our testes to produce more testosterone.

4. Then, through more magic that we don't need to understand or delve into, the Leydig cells in the testicles convert cholesterol into testosterone. They get most of the cholesterol they need to produce testosterone by merely absorbing what's floating around in our blood from the delicious game meats, steak, eggs, and bacon we should be eating on a regular basis. That is, by consuming more fats we **feed our body's ability to produce testosterone. Boom.**

5. The T is now produced and sent back into our bloodstream at which point most of it attaches to SHBG and albumin (two molecules that attach to

testosterone, making this form of T 'bound testosterone) making it biologically inert. **The 2-3% that remains unbound is free to circulate our bodies making us men.**

Note: when the hypothalamus detects that we have enough T in our blood, it signals our pituitary gland to stop secreting LH to diminish our testosterone production. Hence, when you inject a synthetic form of the hormone into your body, your brain tells this production process to halt.

CHAPTER 8

THINGS YOU CAN DO TO BOOST YOUR TESTOSTERONE LEVELS NATURALLY

"There is a constantly reoccurring notion that real manhood is different from simple anatomical maleness, that it is not a natural condition that comes about spontaneously through biological maturation but rather is a precarious or artificial state that boys must win against powerful odds. This recurrent notion that manhood is problematic, a critical threshold that boys must pass through testing, is found at all levels of sociocultural development regardless of what other alternative roles are recognized."

~ David Gilmore

You likely have *one thing* that will make by far the biggest difference, and as we go through the do's and don'ts, it will become apparent what that something is.

Two examples:
1. *Sleep: a quality sleep can do wonders as it will help you lower your cortisol levels dramatically if you're not currently getting enough sleep.*

2. *Lose fat: body fat is incredibly estrogenic. If you're carrying more than 14% body fat, that (along with getting a good sleep) will be the most important thing for you to focus on. Everything else will be secondary.*

In your attempt to create not just good, but optimal testosterone levels, there are things you can do that will help you produce more testosterone and free testosterone, and there are things you shouldn't do that will remove the barriers that are standing between you and this glorious hormone.

Go through both lists. Identify what you aren't doing that you could add to your routine quickly, and the things you are doing that you can stop doing.

Again, the goal is to simplify.

No tricks or magic potions here. **We're simply curtailing your current routine in a way that is easily sustainable, and that will help you produce the optimal testosterone levels you need to be at your best as a man, in life, in bed, in the gym, and so on and so forth.**

Chapter 9
The Do's

"We do not admire the man of timid peace. We admire the man who embodies victorious effort; the man who never wrongs his neighbor, who is prompt to help a friend, but who has those virile qualities necessary to win in the stern strife of actual life."

~ Theodore Roosevelt

1. Don't just go through the motions in the gym.

You may know that exercises that focus on bigger, lower body muscle groups like squats and deadlifts help provide you with a surge in testosterone, and it's true, they do, which is why your program should be dominated by both exercises. But it's not just squats and deadlifts that boost testosterone, things like plyometrics and Olympic lifts do as well.

Here's the thing…

These bigger, more explosive lifts may result in a surge

in testosterone in the moment, but they'll also help you burn more fat in the long run, creating a better atmosphere for testosterone overall in your life as well. You need to maintain as much muscle as you possibly can and focusing on power and strength will help you do that even while you're at a caloric maintenance (when you're consuming as many calories as you're burning), or at a brief caloric deficit (when you're consuming fewer calories than you're burning in the run of a day).

While you get a surge in testosterone from the heavier, explosive compound lift or exercise, you're also having a more significant impact on your muscle mass, and in the world of producing optimal testosterone - and heck, even living an optimal life - having powerful, strong muscle mass is a great ally.

Any workout program should be centered around heavier lifts and the bigger muscle groups. If these aren't at the core of your workout, if you're not doing them at least twice a week (more on this later), you need to change how you're training - and I'll provide more insight into how you should do this later in the book. [1]

2. Compete daily.

Competition isn't just necessary for our development as men. It's not just a matter of success or dominating others; we need it for our health.

Men are born to compete. In fact, we're rewarded hormonally for competing, and again for winning.

Multiple studies have been done on this rise in testosterone in men pre and post competition.[2] When men are about to compete, we experience increased testosterone levels. We then experience another boost when we win in comparison to when we lose.

If you think back to our history as humans, and especially as men, we needed any advantage we could get before we took part in our two primary roles: provider and protector.

That is, we were either in some form of battle, defending our tribe or conquering another, or we were hunting with our primitive tools in lands populated by beasts far bigger, stronger, and deadlier than we were.

Testosterone acted as that reward.

So, as a man, you need to keep competition in your life. As we age, we often lose this, but we need it. Physical competition (sports, especially combat sports) is best.

Join a boxing gym, a BJJ gym, learn how to fight and defend yourself and spar on a regular basis. Feel the elation of victory and the rush of primal competition. Boxing is my favorite form of competition. It's chess with fists. Winning is fantastic, glorious even, and losing is crushing, but the rush of competition is tough to beat in a combat sport where it's just you and your opponent.

The best aspect of combat sports - including boxing, jiu-jitsu, wrestling, and so forth - is that you can continue doing them well into the latter years of your life, especially jiu-jitsu. So find ways to compete, and don't think you're too old to compete on a physical level, you need it.

3. Win.

Winning in any form, be it making money, beating someone up (in a competition), winning a game, winning a lady in a duel, all lead to increased testosterone levels.

BE A WINNER.

In our politically correct society, we're beginning to degrade the necessity for victory to avoid hurting the feelings of those who have not yet won. **We need victory!** We need accomplishment in our lives to feel as though we're here for a reason. What few people ever understand, however, is that **they can define what victory is, you do not have to adhere to your society's or culture's idea of what winning entails.**

You get to make your definition according to what you want in life and who you want to become. BUT, don't diminish the necessity of working your ass off to become that man and to create that life.

To have pride, confidence, happiness, and purpose, you need to have accomplishments.

It'll also boost your testosterone levels.
[3],[4],[5],[6],[7]

When men win, we experience a surge in testosterone. When we have a big financial score, we get a big boost. In a study of stock traders, one trader went on a winning spree and experienced a 78% increase in testosterone. This is powerful, but it won't be talked about in many 'testosterone boosting programs or products' because it asks you to do something more than eat this or that or take this or that, it asks you to hustle, to think, to learn, grow, and evolve as a man.

Whatever you're doing in your life for work, win.

Take winning as seriously as you do your hormones. Invest in yourself. Buy books. Study how to become better at whatever it is that you're doing. I'm going to test this on myself. But I know what the results will be. When I'm winning – and winning is so often a matter of perspective, we're usually winning without really appreciating the fact or acknowledging it – I feel POWERFUL. I feel in charge. I lead. I'm better in relationships. I'm more calm and confident in public.

Define victory and grab that bitch! Do what you need to do to win with honor.

4. Sleep.

Sleep is likely the most important thing you can do to lower your cortisol levels. And, cortisol being one of the two major enemies of testosterone, means that by getting better, longer sleep, this may be the biggest key to unlocking your testosterone-boosting potential.

One study by Penev et al. found that men who slept for ~4 hours had an average of 200-300 ng/dL testosterone levels in serum. Guys who slept for ~8 hours had levels closer to 500-700 ng/dL. Other studies show a decrease in testosterone by 15% when getting only 5 hours of sleep per night for one week. If you're sleeping less than 7 hours a night, this could be the culprit.

At the foundation of your plan to naturally increase your testosterone levels, to get them to your body's optimal levels, you need to ensure you're getting enough sleep - and for the vast majority of us, that means 8 hours.

When I set out to study testosterone, I wasn't sleeping enough. I planned my sleep around an Arnold Schwarzenegger speech where he made the reasoning that we as driven, ambitious men only need 6 hours of sleep a night. I loved the logic. By getting two fewer hours of sleep, I was allowing for two more hours of work a week, which added up to 14 more hours of work every week, which is astronomical!

So, I went to bed later and woke up earlier and my work suffered.

What? I was working more, working longer hours, putting more time in, yet I was getting less work done, and the quality of my work was diminished as well. Why?

Then I came across a series of books that changed my perspective on hours worked versus work done. It started with the *One Thing*, by Gary Keller, and then *Essentialism*, by Greg McKeown. Both books changed the way I viewed my work. They forced me to focus on the most critical tasks first, and only on those tasks. By doing this I was able to get more work done in less time, *much more work* actually, and the quality was much greater. Then I read *Deep Work*, by Cal Newport. Newport introduced other ideas, like adding a deadline, a firm shut down to the workday. This helped me, again, improve the amount of work I got done, and its quality. He also introduced the idea of a 90-minute work block dedicated solely to a single, important task. Each book forced me to say 'no' to more and more opportunities and yes only to the opportunities that would move the needle and dramatically improve business.

I then decided to focus on getting 8 hours of sleep every night by installing a sleep schedule into my routine. As a young fella, I had insomnia - I couldn't sleep for the life of me. Doctors prescribed a bunch of nonsense, and finally, I tried a sleep schedule. That sleep schedule was the only thing that worked. It trained my mind and my body to fall asleep at a specific time, and it worked. Implementing it once again had the same effect.

The contrast in work amount and quality when I'm getting 8 hours of sleep versus 6 hours, is drastic. Never again will I aim to get anything less than 8 hours. Now I know you're likely a driven guy who sees that 14 hours of extra work time a week as an edge over your competition. It isn't.

Getting more sleep and better sleep will help you get more work done, it will help with creativity, and it will help increase your testosterone levels in dramatic fashion.

Set a sleep schedule that you follow every day for the next two weeks. Document how you feel at the beginning, and then again at that two-week mark. You'll notice a difference, and it will improve nearly every other area of your life as well.

5. Have sex and don't watch porn.

It's been studied and proven, but the reasons why sex (and not just watching sex) naturally increase our testosterone levels isn't entirely known.

The studies, though, show massive increases in testosterone in men when they're having sex, or on nights where they know sex is going to occur. So have lots of it. Get off porn and have some damn sex with your lady!

This is just another reason to get off porn. Check out yourbrainonporn.com for more studies on the adverse effects on porn, but one thing that it will do is curb your desires for the visual and away from the physical.

No man in his right mind would want to watch sex more than he wants to have it, yet that's just one of the myriad effects porn has on our brains. To delve deeper into the negative effects, men are here, in part, to procreate.

You need the challenge, the fear, and the possibility of failure that comes with pursuing a lady.

For your personal development, you need to experience this. Those of you who have a lady and want to have more sex, we're going to cover this a bit later both from a mentality standpoint and including a 'cocktail' you can have daily to improve your erection strength and frequency. But sex is paramount; porn is an illusion. Think about your ancestors. Think about the Vikings, the Anglo Saxons, the Romans, or whatever culture you hail from, they were, at some point in time, conquerors. They had a lady, a family. They made babies. They had virility. Now think of a millennial. Even the images we see when we think of our ancestors emasculate the hell out of our current state.

As porn addiction becomes rampant everywhere, as young men learn about sex by watching the perversion of it that exists on the other end of a screen. Do the work of finding a lady. Get that positive and negative feedback. Turn your back on the illusion and seek reality. You'll not only have higher testosterone levels as a result, but you'll be a damn man, not basement dweller.

Three Studies on Sex

1. The first study sent 44 men to a sex club (not kidding). The men who went there to watch sex saw an 11% increase in their testosterone levels. The guys who went there to have sex saw an astonishing 72% increase!

   Meaning, have sex; don't watch sex.[8]

2. In couples, men experience higher testosterone levels on nights when they have sex versus when they don't.[9]

3. In the Baltimore Longitudinal Study on Aging, a famous study that has many more findings than this particular one found that men over 60-years of age who were sexually active had greater serum testosterone levels.[10]

4. Smoke cigars (or at least don't feel horrible about doing it).

Tobacco increases testosterone. The belief is that it does so because it blocks aromatase, much like zinc does, preventing testosterone from being converted into estrogen.

Now, cigars and tobacco pipes aren't 'healthy,' but if you enjoy a cigar from time to time as I do, don't do it with such a weight on your conscience thinking you're destroying your health. You're not. If you have a cigar a week – as per a nose, ear, throat specialist – you're fine (disclaimer, talk to your specialist before taking my advice on this).

The initial study in the book *did note* that one of the things that stood out about the decline in testosterone was also a reduction in smoking. They hypothesized that it may be more about the weight gain that also took place over the period of the study, but it's still interesting – though probably not the best correlation. There could be some (a small ounce) merit to that. However, it seems our increasingly sedentary lifestyle, rise in obesity, and the creation and domination of plastics have had a greater effect on our hormones.[11],[12]

5. Consume a healthy amount of fats (but the right kind).

So, fat (cholesterol) is where we get testosterone. It's how testosterone is produced. We need cholesterol to have testosterone in the first place.

Not all fats, however, are created equal.

Saturated (SFAs) and monounsaturated (MUFAs) fatty acids increase your testosterone levels. Polyunsaturated (PUFAs) and trans-fats suppress the production of testosterone (we're going to cover dietary fats in greater detail in a bit).

For quality fats, animals are your best bet, but specifically game meats. That may not be a 'popular' thing to say as many get their panties in a knot when it comes to hunting, but there's no doubting that the quality of meat from a wild animal is far healthier than one kept in confinement and fed crap its entire life.

If you're inclined, then start hunting. It's the best way

to explore the great outdoors and to connect to what our ancestors did to find food. If you're not inclined, then befriend a hunter or find a butcher who specializes in game meats.

The thing about hunting is that it's not only cheaper, you aid in the conservation of the wildlife you're hunting, ensuring that the next generation will flourish, and you get a great workout while you're out there. [13],[14],[15],[16]

Note: **The correlation between the two healthy fats and heart disease has never been all that strong according to recent research either.**[17]

6. Consume ample amounts of cholesterol.

We have to talk about fats twice because of the misconceptions surrounding them.

For one, having a high cholesterol diet doesn't correlate to high cholesterol levels in the blood over an extended period. Furthermore, the more cholesterol you consume, the less your body has to produce on its own. Increased dietary cholesterol and blood levels of HDL cholesterol (the good kind), positively affect testosterone levels (which makes sense because this is where testosterone comes from).

I would, however, find a good butcher.

I don't eat conventional bacon from the grocery store. Instead, I have wild boar bacon, always paired with free range eggs.

Quality matters.

And again, if you hunt or fish you're going to be ahead of the game for the quality of the food you're consuming. [18],[19],[20],[21]

7. Keep your balls healthy and cool.

As much as 95% or so of the testosterone flowing through your body comes from your testicles.

Hence the necessity to take care of the fellas that are producing the vast majority of your testosterone. Just like you're going to take care of your brain so you can think and learn and earn money (which will boost your testosterone levels), you're going to have to take care of your balls as well.

Temperature is where you're going to do the most good when it comes to testicular health. They need to be cooler than the rest of your body – which is why they dangle in a sack away from the rest of the body when they're hot, but pull themselves closer to the body when they're cold. Thus, wearing 'nut-hugger' underwear or jockeys isn't the greatest thing for your balls, just like those cyclist spandex or riding a bike for hours on end.

This naturally brings up a Seinfeld episode where Kramer is faced with the news that his sperm count is low. The doctors tell him to let his boys breathe, so he tries boxers, but finally settles on 'freeballing,' or wearing nothing but his jeans, which is not a bad idea. I opt for boxers, because of the comfort, but whatever you wear, make sure they give the fellas room to breathe.

A couple of things you can do to ensure testicular health:

- *Take cold showers once or twice a day (also help to make you tougher – I go 5 minutes in the morning and 5 minutes at night as there's evidence that cold showers also help with sleep).*

- *Wear loose boxers instead of tight underwear or boxer briefs.*

- *Sleep naked.*

You essentially want to give them air to breathe.

8. Eat Carbs!

Yes, you have to consume fat to increase your T levels, but study after study has shown that carbohydrates help you increase testosterone as well.

So, carbs...

By diminishing your carbohydrate intake, you're going to wreak havoc on your hormones, and you're going to negatively impact your sleep (which is one of the most critical aspects of this testosterone-boosting adventure you're about to embark upon).

One study found that a diet high in carbs and low in protein leads to 36% higher free-testosterone level and lower cortisol production compared to a diet with high-protein low-carbs [22] (as a caveat, there are other studies that show the importance of protein as it relates to testosterone - which you'll see next - so while some studies push a low-protein diet, you actually need both, especially where body composition is concerned. Protein helps promote a healthy body composition, you need it, but you also need carbohydrates.).

Another study set two groups of men undergoing intensive cycling 3x/week to eat a diet of either 30% energy from carbs or 60% energy from carbs.

It found that the group that eats fewer carbs will have

significantly lower free-testosterone levels. This is powerful and interesting. Not only has there been a war on fat, but a very recent war on carbohydrates, with our view of protein remaining relatively positive, but it's carbs and fats that should exist in a testosterone diet – carbs at around 35% and fats at 35% with calories coming from protein filling the leftover 30%.[23]

Some people thrive on higher fat diets – like myself, as I find myself a bit lethargic on higher carbohydrate diets, but I don't drop beneath that 30% mark. This is something you have to test out yourself. I'm not going to tell you the EXACT number of carbs you should eat because that will fluctuate with how active you are. The more active (a training day) you are, the more carbs you're going to need to consume. I also use my carbs in that I have them during and after a workout, using them to slow the rise of cortisol we experience during a workout, and also helping me fall to sleep by consuming most of them later in the day. I don't have them in the morning or the afternoon because I don't want to mess with my energy levels.

9. Eat Protein.

While there are studies above that show that a high protein, low carb diet is detrimental to your testosterone levels, they don't show that a high protein, high carb, high fat diet is. And sometimes you just have to test things out yourself to find the truth, but you also have to use logic, and logic dictates that with the positive effects of protein on body composition, it's an ally.

After I created a product called the Testosterone

Routine, I went on an anti-protein binge. Study after study 'proved' that protein had a negative effect on testosterone. However, protein spikes insulin, just like carbs do, it's tougher to break down than carbs meaning it has a better effect on your metabolism, and it helps repair tissue just like testosterone does.

That's where we see the biggest benefit of protein, in tissue repair, more specifically helping your muscles recover. You need muscle to be optimally anabolic, meaning, muscle keeps you lean, it keeps your estrogen levels low, allowing your testosterone levels to thrive.

Test things. See how you feel with a lower protein intake, but I need to get at least 30% of my calories from protein, or else my body gains too much fat. I've seen the same happen with a number of clients as well. [24]

10. Drink coffee.

This is interesting…

One study found that 4mg/kg of caffeine taken 1-hour before exercise can increase T levels by 12% (that's pretty insane). Even more interesting are the effects of tea (which I perceived to be a healthier alternative to coffee) on our hormones. Tea that is high in fluoride (green tea) lowers testosterone levels. **Injecting green tea into rodents reduced their testosterone levels by 70%.** The catechins and tannins in various teas have a mechanism of blocking DHT synthesis via reducing 5-a enzyme

It's not what we're told by health gurus, but we should be choosing coffee over tea. Coffee tastes better, and it's better for us. And the amount we can consume on a daily basis is surprising.

As a caveat, when you drink too much, your cortisol levels rise, but they don't stay high. Make sure you're consuming enough of the nutrients that lower cortisol throughout the day (like the nutrients found in the Barbarian Manhood Multi - averagetoalphasupplements.com) to ensure that you blunt this rise. Now...

How much caffeine can you have in the run of a day?

6 mg/kg of body weight.

That's a fair bit.

There are 70mg of caffeine in an espresso, so at my weight of 185 pounds, I can have seven espressos per day without damaging my health (please check me on my math).

If you want to experience testosterone boosting benefits, confine a good portion of your caffeine intake to before your workout.[25],[26],[27],[28]

11. Hydrate.

The two primary enemies of testosterone are cortisol and estrogen. We've covered estrogen a heck of a lot thus far, but cortisol is an equally destructive adversary. Studies show that even a 1-2% dehydration can dramatically increase cortisol levels.

Water doesn't just help improve energy and body function, your muscles are made up of a majority of water, as is your brain, and hydrating correctly can rid your body of the harmful chemicals that increase your estrogen levels that we've already covered.

So how much should you drink?

Consume ¾ to 1 gallon of water a day and add 1 to 1.5 liters on to that per hour of exercise.

I've tested many, many methods for improving energy over the years, and hydrating properly is at the top of that list. But don't just leave your hydration to when you're thirsty. Every day I fill a liter mug of water to the brim, drink it, then repeat 4-5 times throughout the day. I mark off how many I've drunk because I continually forget if I just had a drink or not. Don't leave your water intake to chance. Also, don't drink out of plastic bottles. Use glass or metal. Avoid the chemical estrogens that we'll talk about in a sec by avoiding the containers that feed them into your body like a Trojan Horse. [29]

12. Sprint.

High-Intensity Interval Training (HIIT), or short bursts of intense activity followed by rest and recovery are excellent for testosterone production. They provide intense production of lactic acid without being too long to produce increases in stress hormones.

HIIT can cause sharp increases in total testosterone, free testosterone, DHEA, growth hormone, and dihydrotestosterone. As you'll see in the 'don'ts' section, it's much better to sprint than it is to go for long runs.

With that said, there are things you're going to do that will be easy and beneficial to change, and then there are things that provide you with joy, peace, and clarity, like going for a run may do. So while you're reading this list, begin to think about the things you're willing to do and those you're not willing to do.

I sprint. But I also go for long runs. I love - or hate - going for long runs because of the challenge they provide. They're a test. There are always moments where I want to quit or start walking, and I don't. I push through and continue to run. I also love that runner's high that you get when you're well into a run. So while I know that long runs aren't good for my testosterone levels, these are one of the things that I'm not participating in. You have to pick and choose - or not, do your thing - but it's called the Man Diet in part because guys need and want freedom. We're not going to abide by something that's insanely restrictive. So do the big things, like getting your body fat percentage down, and getting good sleep, and consuming enough dietary fat, and be selective with the smaller things like whether you jog or sprint. Of course, you may love to sprint and hate to jog, in which case you're golden. [30],[31],[32]

13. Choose your produce wisely.

We've talked briefly about Chemical estrogens, and one of the more rampant sources of chemical estrogens are the kind we find on our fruits and vegetables and in the foods that the animals eat that we then eat.

Now, organic produce can be more expensive, and not all pesticides are harmful to your hormones, so you don't have to go nuts with organics.

However...

In Denmark, they've looked at the effect of conventional pesticides on the farmers who spray them, and they've found lowered sex hormones when compared to farmers who produce organic foods whom also have higher sperm quality and sex hormone levels.

Now, this isn't a blanketed statement against pesticides. GMOs have allowed us to feed the poor, to get food to places where they can't get it, to defeat famine, and to even enjoy foods we may not have access to otherwise. GMOs aren't evil, nor are they always bad for your T levels, nor are pesticides.

Wash your food.

Your produce shouldn't be your main concern when avoiding chemical estrogens. Most of your avoidance of chemical estrogens should be focused on plastics and the things you put on your skin like deodorant, shampoo, soap, and so forth.

The best option is to simply choose your seeds and grow your own or befriend a farmer if organics are too expensive. I go either or. Keep in mind that the largest growing sector of the organics market is coming from China, where their practices for growing 'organic' food is horrible, usually far worse than any pesticide-covered apple would be.[33],[34]

At the end of the book, I'll provide a list that you can also download at themandietbook.com, along with other resources, print them out, and post them on your fridge. It'll make things easier to follow.

Chapter 10
Don't

Discipline is the difference between what you want now and what you want most.

THE BATTLE BETWEEN a mediocre you and a great you is waged in your habits. Do the right things and don't do the wrong things.

The same applies to your testosterone levels.

Avoid the following things and you're going to remove some massive roadblocks out of your way.

Each of the things on this list acts like a damn, when you remove them from your life you free your testosterone up to flow freely throughout your body.

1. Don't use products that have these chemicals.

"An endocrine disruptor is a synthetic chemicals or natural substances that may alter the endocrine system (consisting of glands, hormones, and cellular receptors that control the body's internal functions) and may cause developmental or reproductive disorders." You're going to find a lot of these endocrine disruptors in soaps, shampoos, deodorants, plastics, pesticides, preservatives, and other appliances and foods.

This isn't to say you're going to freak out and remove all cleaning products and plastics from your life. You wouldn't be able to live, and there are alternatives.

When you hear that our current society is less conducive to producing actual men, this lends credence to that notion. Everywhere around you there are these endocrine disruptors, chemicals that artificially increase your estrogen levels.

You do not need, nor should you in any way want to, increase your estrogen levels.

In an attempt to send your testosterone levels skyrocketing, you should remove all barriers. We talk - and will talk more - about reducing your body fat percentage to fend of estrogen, as well as getting a good sleep to fend off cortisol, but you're also fighting a daily battle against these chemicals, and they're likely found in your deodorant, shampoo, soap, and the plastics that you carry your food and water in. While I say 'don't freak out', this *is* something that is under your control, **and we're trying to control everything we can while ignoring what we can't.**

You can't control your genetics, but you can control what you carry your water in.

There are also chemicals that you have to watch out for and others that are harmless.

Below is a list of the most important chemicals to watch

out for. Read labels, if you find any of these on products you're going to use regularly, I'll show you other options.

Bad Chemicals Include:

- *Bisphenol A (BPA)*
- *Phthalates*
- *Parabens*
- *Triclosan and Triclocarban*
- *Phthalates*
- *Benzophenones (BP-1, BP-2, BP-3)*
- *Polychlorinated Biphenyls (PCBs)*
- *Also watch out for air fresheners – just flat out avoid them.*

Immediate steps to take:

a. *Use a water filter – a carbon one is more than good enough.*

b. *Avoid plastic, so use glass or steel for your drinking water.*

c. *Buy natural deodorants, shampoos and such.*

2. Don't be a vegan or vegetarian!

I get questions weekly from vegans or vegetarians asking about ways they can naturally boost their testosterone levels. I don't respond to them.

Sure, you can supplement to create more testosterone in your system if you're a vegetarian or vegan, but eating meat has been proven time and time again to be the most effective thing you can do from a diet standpoint to have more testosterone and free testosterone flowing throughout your body. So, I don't deal with guys who don't eat meat. If you're not going to do one of the most important things for your testosterone levels, I'm not going to delve into the tricks you can use to make your way around such a big obstacle.

By removing animals from your diet you're getting in the way of consuming enough cholesterol and saturated fats, the fuel for your testosterone, and you're unlikely to have a balanced amino-acid intake.

We've covered a few things already in the 'do's' section that an all-vegetable diet make very difficult to achieve.

a. *It's difficult to consume enough calories on a vegetarian diet.*

b. *You're going to get more PUFAs and not enough SFAs and MUFAs.*

c. *Your macros – the ratio of energy you get from carbs, fats, and proteins – will be difficult to abide by while eating only veggies.*

d. *The quality of the proteins and fats you get will be diminished in comparison to a diet that has both vegetables, fruits, and meats.*

Many studies have found that plant-based diets create lower testosterone levels.

One study found that changing from a meat-based diet

(keep in mind that they never have the controls to say it's a healthy meat-based diet, they simply categorize meat-eaters as people eating meat, even if it's burgers and beers, and *still*, it's been shown, even with all these flaws in the studies, to be better for men than vegetarian or vegan diets are) to a plant-based diet resulted in a 26% reduction in free testosterone levels which are, again, the kind of testosterone that researchers believe is the most important form – if not the only important form – of testosterone.

Another study found a 36% reduction in total testosterone levels on a plant based diet.

Other studies find that plan-based diets create more SHBG levels and lower free T levels, meaning you could have the same overall testosterone levels on a plant-based diet, but because of the different nutrients provided from a plant-based diet you're going to have more of your testosterone bound to a protein and less able to move freely throughout your body doing what testosterone is supposed to do.

You want to remove as many barriers as possible between you and optimal hormone levels. Adopting a plant-based diet and removing meat from your diet will simply place yet another barrier in front of you.

However, you have to keep in mind that the choice isn't meat or veggies. It's both. A majority of your calories from carbohydrates should come from fruits and vegetables.[35],[36],[37]

To reiterate an important point about these studies…

Vegans or vegetarians decide to go down either path because they *think* it's healthier. That's important. They're making an active decision to choose a seemingly healthier lifestyle. The meat eaters in the study are not necessarily even trying to live a healthier lifestyle, they just have meat in their diets, they also likely consume alcohol (which hurts testosterone), and cheap, bad calories that do no good for the body like refined sugars. And yet they still find that these meat-eaters have higher testosterone levels.

I'd love to see a study done on an all meat diet versus an all vegetable diet. From the case studies I've seen, the all meat diet would blow the veggie eaters out of the water. That, however, has yet to be proven, so we'll hold off on going all meat for now. That said, eat meat! Eat it with every meal. Eat as much of it as you want. Just don't follow a diet high in refined sugars (like sauces) to go along with the delicious animals you're going to consume.

3. Don't restrict calories.

The study below pitted two groups together. Group one ate a caloric deficit and ate lean and clean (1350–2415 kcal/day), and the second group ate a normal western diet. The eat clean and stay fit group had 31% LOWER testosterone levels!

Even though they were 'being healthy', their T levels were beneath the normal, western diet group. Now, we can combine some of these (and we will in our routine) to *feed* our testosterone production rather than our fat stores. This comes from consuming carbs at the right time and proteins and fats at the right time.

But make sure you're eating enough![37]

4. Don't consume too much alcohol.

What you want to avoid is *chronic* consumption of alcohol, not necessarily a wholesale avoidance of the delicious beverages.

One study on rats found a 50% reduction in testicle size with 5% of calories coming from alcohol.

Other studies link chronic alcohol consumption with low T levels and higher estrogen levels.

Now, the studies finding that alcohol lowers testosterone levels are focused on alcoholics and chronic consumption. There's little evidence that moderate consumption of alcohol has any significant effect. In fact, one study found that 0,5g/kg of alcohol actually slightly increased testosterone levels.

Thus, it isn't the booze, but the amount you drink. If you're a weekly drinker of scotch, beers, or wine, you're fine. If you drink every day in excess, you're fucked.

Does the kind of alcohol matter?

Yes, basically with beer. Beer is the most estrogenic of the kinds of alcohol you'll consume. Still, you have to be abusing it to have a *real* negative effect on your hormones. If you're going to drink it's better to choose whiskey or wine. I obviously drink (if you follow my site, instagram, or Facebook accounts you'll know this). I rarely *get drunk*, though. I enjoy a drink or two or three every now and then like I enjoy cigars, in moderation. [38],[39],[40],[41],[42]

5. Don't eat these foods.

What I ideally want to do with the *Man Diet,* is to simplify the hell out of this quest to walk around with consistently high testosterone levels.

High estrogen levels in men are always directly related to low testosterone levels in men.

We've talked about a couple things that you can do, including dropping your body fat levels, avoiding pesticides, but there are also foods you should simply avoid all-together. As a basis, don't eat the following:

- *Green Tea*

- *Soy products*

- *Mint, spearmint, peppermint (including in gum, mints, and in your drinks)*

- *Liquorice*

- *High-PUFA vegetable oils*

- *High-PUFA nuts*

- *Flaxseed products*

- *Trans-Fats*

- *Alcohol (I don't avoid this completely, obviously, but opt for whiskey as often as possible over beer)*

6. Don't jog.

We went over this briefly in the do's section, but I wanted to fire you a few more studies, and to drive home the fact that this is actually something I choose to do even though I know it's not great for my testosterone levels. I actually run a fair bit and it's not something I'm going to stop doing even though the science is against prolonged endurance training.

The evidence shows that endurance runners – who are extremely healthy and fit – have even lower testosterone levels than their sedentary counterparts in the studies.

That seems crazy, but it's completely due to the increases in cortisol that you experience during prolonged, intense exercise.

With that said, this is your choice.

If you take care of everything else on this list, you're probably going to be fine running a few times a week. It's not something I'm going to stop doing, but if you have low testosterone levels as a result of high cortisol levels, and you're a runner, it's not a bad idea to switch to sprints, walking, or hiking.

Both walking and hiking keep the heart rate low enough so as to avoid those cortisol spikes that reduce testosterone levels. While I do run, I do it a few times a week, and I walk every day (or hike).[43],[44]

7. Don't slouch!

I remember watching her TED talk years ago. It made me completely rethink how I carried myself, how I sat, walked, talked, and presented myself. It's not a change in who you are, but sitting and standing and *being* powerful in your posture can have a powerful impact on your hormones.

Her name, of course, is Dr. Cuddy. You can check out her TED talk here for yourself (highly recommend it):

https://www.youtube.com/watch?v=Ks-_Mh1QhMc

Her findings are incredible.

After only 2-minutes of 'power-posing' subjects saw a 20% increase in salivary testosterone levels, and a 25% decrease in cortisol – that infamous stress hormone that opposes testosterone.

The opposite was true for slouching, or sitting in a weak position (arms or legs crossed signifying a lack of confidence, for example), where subjects saw a decrease in T and a rise in cortisol.

Having correct, powerful posture is a simple thing you can do that can make a very big difference in your testosterone production.

Surprisingly, in 2-minutes power-posing led to 20% increase in salivary testosterone levels, and -25% decrease in the stress hormone; cortisol. On the contrary, low-power posing led to a drop in T with accompanied rise in cortisol.

CHAPTER 11
THE DAILY TESTOSTERONE ROUTINE

"Excellence is an art won by training and habituation. We do not act rightly because we have virtue or excellence, but we rather have those because we have acted rightly. We are what we repeatedly do. Excellence, then, is not an act but a habit."

- Aristotle

WE'VE GONE OVER a bunch of different tips and tools to help you boost your testosterone levels, we've also covered things you *shouldn't do* as well (which are just as important).

The previous part of this book has been the *why*. Next is the what.

The *why* is as necessary as the *what*. It gives you clarity as to why you're doing what you're doing and without clarity we're unlikely to follow what's laid out for us.

Now, however, you know why we're going to do some

things and not do other things, so we're able to lay out the routine for you and you can simply follow it.

Now, this routine may not reflect your schedule, and that's not a problem.

Within each thing you're doing you're going to be told why it's there. The post workout shake, for example, is to be consumed after the workout. The post workout meal is the same. The other meals stay on the periphery of the workout. On non-workout days you can have the shake and the meal whenever you like, though I like to consume both as my last meals so as to use the insulin spike that carbohydrates provide to slow down and have a better sleep.

As far as the ingredients, they can be swapped as well. You have a carb, swap it for another carb, or a fat, do the same.

In the routine I'll give you other examples, but it won't be a long list. The more options we have, the more we're set aback by information overload, allowing our *current* habits to take over.

Sleep.

Before you start thinking about adopting a nutritional framework (which both I and Stephen Anton, a leading researcher in the realm of intermittent fasting - a tool we'll be using to create optimal T and HGH levels, while staying lean) create a sleep schedule.

You may not *want* to do this, but it's the most important factor in creating consistently good, deep, and healthy sleep. With this daily routine - and the diet - we're tackling testosterone's enemies. While you need dietary fats to fuel your T levels, they won't get very far if there are barriers stacked up in front of them. You need to break down the barriers - namely cortisol and estrogen - if you're going to open the floodgates and see those T levels thrive, not just survive.

The quality and quantity of your sleep is incredibly important. It will not only help your testosterone levels by reducing your cortisol levels, but you're going to be a happier, more productive guy.

The cycle of destruction that a lack of sleep brings into our lives is dangerous. The actual *act* of not getting enough sleep increases cortisol, but the cloudiness and the lack of clear-thinking that results from sleep-deprivation has the same effect.

Much of the stress in our lives is a matter of perspective, and when we're not thinking clearly, we pile it on by worrying about things that are out of our control. By getting a good quality sleep you're combating cortisol in more than one way.

Take a look at your day and create a schedule that you follow *every day*.

Wake up at the same time every single day of the week. The quality and quantity of your sleep is imperative to you creating optimal testosterone levels. This is us *killing* testosterone's enemies.

You've already learned that cortisol is one of two of testosterone's main enemies or roadblocks standing in the way of you and your *thriving* T levels. A quality sleep goes a *long way* in getting cortisol out of the way.

If I could suggest something (and this has nothing to

do with testosterone, but everything to do with *winning*, which is a big aspect of creating optimal T levels, so maybe it does), RISE EARLY.

Winners rise early.

It's not a set-in-stone rule, but if you look at athletes, CEOs, entrepreneurs, and winners in general, getting up early is a commonality among all of them. I've been reading about winners throughout history for a decade (not all that long, I know, but I have a good few books under the ol' belt) and without exception, be it Robert E. Lee, Theodore Roosevelt, or Napoleon Bonaparte, rising early (by 0600h or earlier) is a constant.

A few more tips for creating optimal sleep:

a sleep schedule is by far the most important thing.

a. *No screens at least an hour before bed. Get that artificial light away from your eyeballs before you're heading to bed.*

b. *No booze after 5 pm – booze may make you lethargic, but they greatly diminish the quality of your sleep reducing your REM sleep. Keep the booze to the late afternoon or early evening at most.*

c. *Carbs at night? If you workout at night, don't shy away from carbs after your workout, they'll be 'used', and that spike in insulin will help you fade to sleep.*

However, it's all moot if you don't have a sleep schedule. This is coming from a lifelong insomniac who went to two sleep doctors who prescribed everything from pills to a light I would keep with me in class in high school and basically wherever I went (the idiots actually thought this was a viable option).

The sleep schedule is the only thing that has **guaranteed a consistent quality of sleep.**

Morning: Rise Early, Boost Early, Boner Early.

We've gone over the necessity of rising early. While the *The Man Diet* will provide tips, tricks, and lifestyle choices to help you boost your testosterone levels, the more you win, the more you'll get surges of testosterone, and let's call a spade a spade, you want to boost your testosterone levels *so you can win!*

Keep in mind that 'winning' is defined by you, not by society or your folks or family, but by you, the man.

The boost comes in the form of a cholesterol surge that takes advantage of the 4am-6am time frame where our bodies produce the most testosterone throughout the day.

Now, if you're on an intermittent fasting protocol (which is all good), we're going to give that its own section in a bit, it'll be written by Steve Anton, a researcher I've teamed up with to bring more value to the intermittent fasting portion of the book and to provide a lot more evidence as well as content than I can provide on the topic.

With this surge of cholesterol we're also going to be working on blood flow.

Now, testosterone is a *yuge* aspect of our manliness. *It is* manliness at its core, basic, most primal level, and so is our ability to function sexually.

You may be fine in that department, but statistically,

you're highly likely to experience some form of failure in the realm of erections over your life. Much of that can be due to low T, which is what we're covering in this routine, but it can also be due to decreased blood flow.

Much of what we'll implement from this book will help in this area, but the cocktail below - which we'll explain in more detail later in the 75 foods section - will help.

The Boner Cocktail

We're going to dive deeper into sex drive and how to optimize it later in the book, but for now you want to have the Boner Cocktail inserted into your day at some point (ideally in the morning or at night to take advantage of your 'testosterone window'). That said, if you're intermittent fasting (more later), you're not going to want to consume anything while you're on a fast. So while it calls for this in the morning, if you're fasting in the morning, take this at night or when your fast breaks, with your first meal - this will all make sense in a bit.

Have *at least* a prescribed serving of each of the following - you'll see the dosage of each later in the book as far as the studies, but for now just use the prescribed dosage on each bottle (this is also a disclaimer, I use at least double, but you can choose either way):

Ginseng
Citrulline
Pycnogel
Garlic Extract

As I write this I'm working on getting a formula close to this - with a couple extra bonuses - in supplement form so you don't have to get each ingredient on its own (which can be tough and expensive). Depending on when you're reading this, it may already be live on averagetoalphasupplements.com.

Testosterone SURGE Cocktail

2 whole, hardboiled eggs (healthy cholesterol)
Zinc (blocks the precursor to estrogen)
3 Brazil nuts
Whole, raw milk (or skim milk if you can't get raw milk)
MCT Oil

The boner cocktail (I couldn't come up with a better name) both directly helps erections (ginseng) and helps your erections and their strength and duration through improved blood flow.

The testosterone surge cocktail is simple, it gives you a surge of cholesterol in the morning and it combats estrogen by inhibiting aromatase, which is responsible for converting testosterone to estrogen (which is a big problem among men).

Both set you up for a day where you *thrive*.

What if you eat breakfast right away?

I'm not a big morning eater. I make my 'breakfast' around 11am, and I wake up at 5am. This cocktail suits me.

If, however, you eat breakfast right away, or if you workout in the morning, we'll cover that now.

No AM Workout
Testosterone Morning Routine

Your workout time will dictate your diet and how you take advantage of your carbohydrates and *lean proteins*.

We've already talked about carbs being *good*, and on non-workout days you can have them whenever you like. You can have them with every meal if you want, I just prefer to lump them into the same meal. You simply want to hit your macros for the day and eat healthy, high quality foods.

Let's say you workout in the evening, what should you do in the morning, and should you be doing any physical activity even though you train at night? Yes!

Do something.

Movement is important. Even though you're not a morning workout guy, that doesn't mean you can't do anything active first thing.

My recommendation is to do push-ups, sit-ups, chin-ups if you can, and go for a walk, then get started with your work day.

The start to your day will, ideally, look like this:

1. Rise, Testosterone and Boner cocktails.

2. Read/journal – this is important for your cortisol levels. Plan your day either the night before or the day of, and stick to the plan. It's a great stress remover. It will help you get more work done.

It will help you step into the day with the right mind-frame, reading helps as well.

3. Eat a meal that's high in fats and protein.

4. Kick some ass.

Reading and reviewing your journal is vital. We'll touch briefly on how to set up your best day in this book. Cortisol is a dangerous hormone that's triggered by stress. Stress is often triggered by perspective, thus, by starting every day by reviewing your plan (you should set your plan at the end of the previous work day, don't start a day without a plan), you understand what must get done. When you *don't* have a plan to your day, chaos ensues. In the battle between what you want now and what you want most, if you don't have a plan, what you want now wins - and that guarantees that you *won't win*.

In my journal I also keep a gratitude section where I write down 3 things I'm thankful for over the past 24 hours. I write that list at the end of every day, but I review it at the beginning. Stress is good. You need stress, you need to take on more than you think you can handle, to accomplish something. Worry, is not.

You're a man, the man. You're on *the Man Diet* for shite's sake! You cannot be a worrier, you must be a warrior. Warrior's see life as a series of challenges they have to rise above. Worriers fear the unknown. Not only is that dumb, but it's a great way to send your cortisol levels through the roof.

Getting a good, calm, purposeful start to your day like

the once prescribed will help. I also recommend taking a couple *Barbarian Manhood Multi* tablets that you can find on averagetoalphasupplements.com. They have an energy blend that's awesome, but they also have your daily intake of vitamin C, which also combats cortisol.

What if you *do* workout in the morning?

AM Workout
Testosterone Morning Routine

So, if you workout in the AM, by all means begin your day with the Testosterone and Boner Surge Cocktails, then train, then have a shake, then have a meal high in carbs about 1-2 hours thereafter.

Your morning will look like this:

1. Testosterone and Boner Cocktails (and Barbarian Manhood Multi)
2. Workout
3. Post Workout Shake
4. Post Workout Carbs Meal

We've gone over the cocktails.

Now, what should you do for your workout?

We'll discuss that next. It doesn't matter if you're training in the morning, afternoon, or evening, your workout will ideally include what's covered next.

The Testosterone Workout

Your workout should include programs and exercises that both in the short term and in the long term help you boost your testosterone levels. In the long term this will mean a reduced body fat percentage and a healthy amount of strong, powerful muscle. In the short term you'll focus on exercises that provide a surge in testosterone as well as the lean muscle mass that your body needs to be optimal.

Now, are surge's important? Yes! Sure, we're trying to create long-term increases in testosterone, but the surge you get from competing, from winning, from making money and performing some of the exercises below are just as important. As you age and become more sedated (this doesn't have to be you), men experience fewer of these surges that we experienced when we were grabbing life by the horns and having our way with it. That aggressiveness, that assertiveness and daring that is usually relegated to youth needs to continue.

Long Term T Boosting Through Training

Working out does *a lot* for your hormones. Long-term, lowered body fat will also lower your estrogen levels, allowing your testosterone levels to thrive.

The *act* of working out boosts your testosterone levels.

One study found that sedentary men experienced a very significant boost in their baseline testosterone levels after starting a resistance-training program. Another study found that the subject's testosterone levels increased by a whopping 40% after only 4 weeks of working out. [44]

Why?

It's likely because our bodies and our hormones have to adapt to the new demands being placed upon them.

Thus, with a program like I'll describe below, you want to continually be improving and pushing yourself to get stronger without hitting a plateau due to inefficient or unintelligent training.

Plateaus can signal over-training, which can signal your cortisol levels being too high, which means you need to take *a little* time off, fully recover, or you need to learn how to *better recover, or* you need to switch up your program. But, the right program will constantly be changing for you so you don't have to do any of that work.

Short Term T-Boosting Through Training

There are exercises that also boost your testosterone levels. Deadlifts and squats, and variations of each, provide a surge in your testosterone levels. As do Olympic lifts, plyometrics, and sprints.

A workout program needs both the long-term benefits of training, the muscle gains, the fat loss, the improvements in posture and so forth, to be an effective program *for testosterone.*

… But you also have other goals in mind, I'm guessing, and that program should ideally fulfill those goals as well.

Here's what that should look like:

The Testosterone Workout Program

A workout that helps you increase your testosterone levels in the long term and in the short term should include these 3 factors:

1. **A strength/muscle-building program that focuses on lifting heavy, activating as much muscle as possible (focuses on the bigger muscles), and progressively helps you improve.**

    Muscle is your greatest ally. It will increase your metabolism. It helps you live a stronger life. But the means by which you get there (focusing on bigger lifts and bigger muscle groups with heavier weights) also give you a *surge* in testosterone, helping you recover faster and recruit more fat cells for fuel, which helps you burn more fat, which helps you lower your estrogen levels.

    A study out of the University of Alabama at Birmingham pitted strength training against endurance and higher-rep training to see which would help the subjects burn more fat.

    You're a guy. You don't want to be a scrawny twig. You also don't want to be round and fat. Muscle is your friend. **Your goal should never be 'weight loss', but fat loss.**

    That's an important distinction. Both methods in the study created the same weight loss. Strength training, however, saw dramatically more *fat loss*. Meaning, strength training helps you burn more fat while also helping you build muscle.

    I've been lifting weights since I was in high school. I've been in this industry for over a decade. Going to the gym and *lifting weights* is not the best way to go about your training.

You will not get the BEST results if you just head to the gym and 'workout'.

Now, we're talking about framework.

That's all that a workout program is. It gives you the framework to guide you to your goal.

We've already talked about the overall method to get to the goal. It doesn't matter if you want to burn fat, build muscle, get stronger, or become a better athlete, strength should be the basic focus (where athletics are concerned, #2 and #3 of this list that a testosterone routine should include will be something you want to look at, as well as substituting some of the bigger exercises with Olympic lifts).

Where strength and building lean, athletic muscle is concerned, there's one method (or framework) that appears to work better than the rest.

This method is called Daily Undulating Periodization.

It's just a bit better than other methods or frameworks (and it's been proven to be so) for a couple reasons.

a.   *It's based on how strong you are.*

   So you start off by determining your 1 rep max in a few important exercises. You determine this number based on math, not based on lifting the heaviest possible weight you can lift (which can be dangerous). From there you determine exactly what weight you should choose for every exercise in the program.

   This is yuge.

You can now walk into the gym knowing exactly what weight you should be lifting. This provides both guidance, and a challenge. Too often we choose a lighter weight based on how we're feeling.

You also know where you are in relation to where you want to be. It's a powerful, mathematical, scientific approach to training.

Fortunately, you don't have to do any math. I've done it all for you. You simply plug your results of the Guage Workout (a 1 week workout to help you determine your strength levels) into the calculators I provide to determine exactly what weight to choose for each exercise.

You can get your free Gauge Workout at themandietbook.com.

b. *It's not pure heavy lifting.*

This is important to avoid over-training. Undulating periodization rotates between intensity (a weight closer to your 1RM) and volume (a lighter weight done with higher reps creating an overall greater weight lifting).

Example:

5 sets of 5 reps for 200 lbs = 5,000 lbs

4 sets of 10 reps for 150 lbs = 6,000 lbs

This helps you see continual growth without experiencing

over training or plateaus (where your body adapts to the weights and exercises you're performing and your improvement hits a plateau).

These two main factors, that you're getting stronger, more powerful, and more muscular, while avoiding plateaus, avoiding our natural tendencies to be lazy (or even to over-do it), make the DUP method ideal.

However, the DUP method on its own isn't the best form of training for your testosterone levels. You still need two other factors.

2. Plyometrics and Olympic Lifts.

The testosterone surge's from training come not only in the bigger, heavier lifts that activate your bigger muscles, but also in explosive movements like plyometrics and Olympic lifts.

If you feel safe doing them, they (or at the very least, sprints) should be a part of your training routine.

I added a lot of both plyometric training and Olympic Lifts so as to gain power without bulk. I added up adding a ton of power, explosiveness, and what seemed like a more dense muscle. If you don't know how to perform either, hire a personal training or an Olympic lifting coach to show you the ropes. Technique is incredibly important, especially with Oly lifts. So spend a couple bucks, learn how to perform them properly, then get after it.

3. Sprints.

In the do's and don'ts I talked about how longer bouts of intense cardio – be it running or biking – has a pretty dramatic effect on your cortisol levels.

I also mentioned how I love to run – well, I don't 'love it', it's painful, which is why I like it. There's always a moment in a run (or many moments) when you'd rather quit than carry on.

Hormonally, however, sprints are a much better alternative.

Creating Your Own Program

With all I've laid out, you can definitely create your own program.

Ideally follow a DUP protocol. Add in Oly lifts and plyometrics, and do some form of sprint training every week, ideally a few times a week.

Or, you can do the one I've already created for you. Just visit themandietbook.com/workout and check it out.

CHAPTER 12

KEEPING OPTIMAL TESTOSTERONE LEVELS DURING THE DAY

*"Winning takes precedence over all.
There's no gray area. No almosts."*

~ Kobe Bryant

YOU'VE ALREADY GONE through a litany of things you can do to both naturally boost your testosterone levels and things you should avoid so as to *allow* your body to produce testosterone optimally.

Toward the end of this book I've put it all in checklist form so you can check either the do's or don'ts off as you go through your day. There are, however, other things to remember before we get into how you end your day.

Also, we haven't even touched on *how* you're going to eat yet. So implement the following, and then add in your *Man Diet* as you see fit, and as it fits your schedule.

Compete. Improve.

We got into this in the do's section, but it's important to reiterate. Men need competition. We need daily improvement.

I get *a lot* of questions about women, how to get them, keep them, lead them, and so forth. I'm not an expert on women, but I know enough to guide guys in the right direction simply from my own experiences.

Women want what you want for yourself.

That is, women want a guy who's getting after it, who has a purpose above and beyond them. They don't want a pleaser. They don't want a guy who will do everything for them. They want a guy who's hustling who wakes up and competes.

That's probably who you want to be as well.

So make a quick list of the things that encompass the guy you have to be to attract your ideal lady.

Leader, warrior, smart, driven, ambitious, in shape, takes pride in how he carries himself, and so on.

If mere self-improvement doesn't drive you to compete day in and day out, then maybe a beautiful lady will. Improving as a man, every day, is competing.

You can also join a team. Join a gym. Learn to fight (which will help with confidence in a big way).

Don't, however, forget that you're here to make the most out of your days. Spending your life as a worrier, as a lost, timid soul is no way to live.

You need to wake up every day with a purpose, on purpose, and headed toward improvement. You need to *end* every day having done something that brings you closer to your ideal, whatever that thing is. You know what your ideal is, your ideal life, your goal. Accomplish at least one thing in a given day that brings you closer to that dream. A good woman doesn't want a lapdog, a 'yes man', and nor should you aspire to be one. The kind of man you are attracts the kind of lady you'll find. Forget about the woman. You have to have your shit together for your own journey. You have to be responsible, self-reliant, and driven in some way. In short, you have to be a man! You must grow up. You cannot remain a child like so many in our society choose to do well into their thirties and forties.

Stand; don't sit.

One theory behind the decline in testosterone in men over the past few decades is that our lives are becoming increasingly sedentary.

We're at a point, as humans, where we're sitting more than ever.

Simply by standing you're going to improve your posture and waistline. There's other evidence that shows a powerful stature or posture helps men have higher testosterone levels.

Slouching caused by sitting too much is the enemy of testosterone. If you're at a desk a lot I *highly* recommend getting a standing desk or adding an apparatus that enables you to stand or sit – this is what I use: http://amzn.to/2tmoFD0.

Move.

Movement, not just standing instead of sitting, is also very important. We discussed being active in the list of do's and how it results in higher testosterone levels in men.

Activity is found in simple choices in your day, like taking the stairs, doing your own yard work, running, walking, or biking to work. Move more; be seated (even in your truck) less.

Humans are not meant to be sedentary. The invention of the seat was one of our species' most destructive. Before its inception all we had was the ground, thus, we stood more, ran more, walked more, hunted more, and many believe that we were a *heck of a lot* healthier as a result.

Breathe Deeply.

Cortisol is an enemy of testosterone, and much of our cortisol can be regulated by our bodies and minds without having to do a ton of changes to our lifestyle or diet (though both will definitely help).

Breathing deeply is a big one. A few times a day spend a minute breathing deeply. Control your breath. Three seconds in, four seconds out.

Short breaths and panting can have the opposite effect, and if you've ever paid attention to your breathing when you're stressed in the middle of a workday, that's likely just what you're doing.

Be aware of your body, how you're thinking, and how you're breathing, and slow down. To add to breathing deeply, breathe into your belly, not your chest. Pay attention to how you're breathing when you're stressed, worried, and feeling the pressure that can come with being the man, you're likely breathing through your chest. That is, the air you're breathing in is going into your chest and not your belly. There's much more space when you set out to breathe through your belly. Try it.

Next time you feel stressed or anxious or worried, stop, relax, and breathe deeply through your belly.

Don't Worry.

Be a warrior, not a worrier. Don't pity yourself. Don't fret over the things that have not yet happened.

The best way I deal with worry is to simply be fearless. I say the word over and over in my head, like a mantra, and I'm able to not worry about things that are out of my control – which is what we primarily worry about.

Worry is the vehicle for cortisol. It's how we become overrun by negative stress (there is good stress in the form of our desire to win and achieve and improve). Worry has no purpose. It has no benefit. Why would you bring something on that does not benefit you in any way? It makes no sense to worry, I think we all understand this, but actually *avoiding it* is something entirely different and more difficult. I'd love to write a book entirely about not worrying, for now, though, read the following:

Man's Search for Meaning, by Viktor Frankl
How to Stop Worrying and Start Living by Napoleon Hill
Meditations by Marcus Aurelius
The Lost Art of Discipline by Chad Howse

Use Your Journal

Cortisol is as much about your perspective, how you deal with stress and how you look at your life and where you're going, as it is a matter of any external force.

We've already talked about planning and setting out the course for your day as well.

Journaling should be a part of your routine, but use your journal for 3 things.

1. Plan your day.

Without a plan for our day we're far more likely to fall victim to our desires in the moment. Planning your day enables you to focus only on the task at hand. There is no guessing. There is no stress about what should or should not be done. You're simply following your day's plan.

Determine the single most important task, and give that task your best hours (the hours where you're best able to focus and produce quality work - for me it's the morning hours).

Then figure out one or two more important tasks and give them your next important hours. Give your time slots blocks, where there's only a single focus.

If that focus isn't work, you should still give it a block so you have a purpose to what you're doing and you're not going to be pulled in many different, stressful and unproductive directions.

At the day's end, check off everything you did.

Your business and time journal should be filled in the night before. Your days should be planned and purposeful. Don't let the stress of 'being busy' get in the way of both the work that must be done or your testosterone levels. Being busy isn't being productive. Plan your day.

2. Thoughts.

A journal should help you find clarity.

To see issues we face in the correct way, we have to detach. We have to look at the problem without the emotions we've attached to it.

Writing an issue down and then solving it on paper helps you calm down, de-stress, and find clarity. I do this daily from business to relationships and it helps me figure out solutions and even just avoid worrying about outcomes when I'm able to write it down and read it for what it is – at most, a minor bump in the road.

3. Outlook.

This is a must.

At the end of every day, write down 3 things you're grateful for that happened within the past 24 hours. It forces you to look for the positive, to see the opportunity, and it allows you to end your day on a positive note, without the stress and worry running through your mind that can negatively affect your sleep.

Your days should be clear and focused and not clouded by worry and stress. While this is *the Man Diet*, it also has to be *the man lifestyle*, for what's the point of increasing your testosterone levels if you're going to piss them away with worry and laziness?

You're the man. Get after it. You don't have time to be worried.

Chapter 13
The Testosterone Evening

"A man must stand erect, not be kept erect by others."

~ Marcus Aurelius

If you workout in the evening, have an awesome workout and make sure you wind down before bed.

It's the winding down that's most important.

You need to set yourself up for a good sleep, but you also need to have a different compartment to your post-work life, *and you should have a post-work life*.

We'll cover a couple things you can do to de-stress, clear your mind, and get as much out of your post-work hours as you do from your working hours. One benefit you have with *the Man Diet* is that carbs come later on in the day. One thing that dietary fats and meats have is that they slow the rise in blood sugar, helping you experience increasing energy levels throughout the day. Carbs and lean proteins, however, increase insulin, which combats cortisol while also giving you a brief spike in energy, but then the 'carbs crash' thereafter.

Having carbs later in the day have helped me wind down in a big way while also helping me improve my sleep quantity and quality.

3 Things you're grateful for that happened in the last 24 hours.

Doing this at the end of every work day or every day is powerful. It sets you up to have an abundance mindset, not one where you're a victim.

End work at the same time every day.

Getting enough work done is rarely about time, and more often a matter of focus. This book isn't about being effective or efficient in your work, but I have written one that will help you *immensely* in your ability to work and win.

Check it out here: **thelostartofdiscipline.com**

By ending work at the same time every day, you make your work more urgent.

Right now, for example, I'm in my backyard writing, and my girlfriend is coming over at 5pm, at which time we'll work on my backyard and take the pup out.

That firm end means I have to have everything I set out to do during the day completed. That urgency forces me to choose what I should focus on more strictly.

You should always only have one thing to focus on. When my lady comes over, it's her and the work we're doing on the yard.

Ending work firmly, rather than allowing it to linger into the night, will also improve your sleep quality.

Don't have caffeine 6 hours before bed

Caffeine, as we've already discussed, is great for your hormones if you have it in the right amounts, if you go over, then it will increase your cortisol levels, if you have it too *late*, it can ruin your sleep.

Cut it off 6 hours before your set bedtime.

Carbs are okay at night if you train at night

As previously mentioned, carb's aren't actually bad at night, especially if you've just worked out and they're going to be used to fuel your muscles and recovery.

Carbs can also help you fall asleep.

The spike in insulin that comes from consuming carbs can knock you out. So if you're training in the evening, you're all good to have your carbs backloaded after the workout.

Turn off the TV at least an hour before bed

If you have a family, *be with them*, not in front of the TV. TV *can be* a great way to wind down once the wee ones are in bed, but a book would be much better.

The blue light that emanates from a TV or computer screen diminishes your sleep quality.

I've given a few books in this document that you can get that are very helpful, there are a bunch more in the Lost Art of Discipline that I gave you a link to earlier.

CHAPTER 14
THE MAN DIET

*"Contemporaries appreciate the man rather
than the merit; but posterity will regard
the merit rather than the man."*

~ Charles Caleb Colton

Alpha

It wasn't long ago that I was walking through a town in Argentina after having come down from a mountain. To get back to where I was staying my aunt and I walked through the huts that bordered the town.

Before the 3-month trip to South America I'd thought about getting a dog. I'd been travelling for nearly a year and I thought a dog would help me settle down a bit, build a home base, focus. Me being me, I didn't just want any dog, I wanted what I thought was the best dog. Initially that was a Cane Corso. With my mom being from Italy, I was intrigued by the breed's history, coming from the dogs that the Romans used in war. Then the Rhodesian Ridgeback caught my eye. Dubbed the 'Navy SEAL' of dog breeds, it's fast, agile, and still powerful.

It was on this walk through the poor part of town after the long hike up the mountain that I was thrown a curveball.

We were walking down a street, I'd expressed some interest in a breed called the Dogo Argentino, but you don't see many of them. Up to this point I'd seen a bundle of Corso's, a few Ridgebacks, but I'd never come across a Dogo. As we're trotting down the mountain, through a slum, or a poor neighborhood - whatever you want to call it - my aunt stopped me, pointed to my left, and looking me in the eye was a massive Dogo standing against a fence. We made eye contact. He growled. I got the hell out of there.

A couple days later we went horseback riding and came upon a group of dogs. One was a Corso, the others were big too. Out of nowhere a Dogo sprinted out of his yard and sent all of the other dogs running.

This is a cool breed. Bred for boar and cougar hunting, they're insanely powerful, fast, and they have the endurance to go on a long hunt.

I began talking to breeders in Argentina and took one fella out for a beer. In his description of the dog and its temperament, I knew I found the breed I wanted.

He likened it to a male lion, the leader of a pride, unconcerned with most everything going on around him except viable threats. The breed is calm, even lazy, unless they need to be otherwise. Teddy, my dogo Argentino has proven to be just that, but a heck of a lot more hyper. My house has big windows at its front, and if any animal or human that Teddy hasn't met walks in front of our house he goes nuts.

This is the same effect that testosterone has on the male psyche. We're rewarded when we win, receiving an influx of testosterone. But we're also punished when we lose, as our production of testosterone declines and our production of cortisol is increased.

Testosterone may also help us focus more effectively. Other studies have shown that both surgeons and chess players receive a big spike – up to 500% - in testosterone before they perform. Life is competition, whether you want to believe it is or not, you're competing for status, for pay, for a lady, for the life you want to lead, and testosterone is your ally in said competition.

Testosterone also makes us more prone to risk. Whereas low testosterone makes us less likely to risk. This is incredibly important.

Throughout our history as a species it's those who've done what others weren't willing to do who have shaped our society. In your own life if you're unwilling to face your fears, to step outside of your comfort zone, you're not going to perform anywhere near your capability. If you shy away from conflict you'll never step into the arena of life. If you persistently choose safety over danger you're never going to rise above the monotonous existence that we've created for ourselves in a society where nearly everything is controlled, and testosterone plays a role in this ability to face danger, fear, risk, and to come out victorious.

The alpha male in a tribe of men or a pride of lions will have more testosterone flowing through his veins than will his second in command or third in command. Winning increases testosterone and testosterone helps you win.

So while this book is a 'how to' on natural production of testosterone through diet and exercise and lifestyle, it would be incomplete without mentioning this, that men who want to live small, inconsequential lives don't really need it. Winners, adventurers, warriors, and leaders, do.

I'm guessing you bought this book because you're more of the latter, or at least you want to be.

I'm going to show you how to burn more fat and build more muscle and ward off depression and disease by naturally increasing your testosterone levels, I'm also going to show you how to win. You're a man, bred from warriors, defenders, and conquerors. You are not meant to live a sedated existence. You cannot be confined to a zoo, you must run wild.

Chapter 15
How Your Current Diet is Ruining Your Masculinity.

- **Have you noticed it more difficult to burn fat than you once could?**
- **Do you find it hard to build lean muscle mass?**
- **Are you suffering from low motivation, low energy, and even depression?**

Low testosterone could be at the root of your problems, and your diet will have a big impact. Even if you're "eating healthy", you may be eating in a way that destroys the most important hormone in your body.

Most diets, as you may know, are created for women. Why? Well, think about it like this...

The fat guy is often content with being fat, drinking beer, and eating his flapjacks every morning, while the thin woman, who by all accounts is walking around at the perfect weight, is far more conscious of what she eats, and how she looks.

Women, on the whole, care about their appearance more than men do. They're more health conscious, and they're more willing to open their wallets to buy a diet, a book, or a guide telling them how to lose fat and flatten their belly.

I'm *in* this industry. All of the products and promotions that occur, that make the most money are focused on helping women lose weight and burn fat. They're emotional about their weight, and emotion sells.

Men don't *care*, nor do they *buy* like women do.

Does that, however, mean that we should be forgotten and relegated to a diet that isn't at all meant for us?!

Ahem. Hell. No.

This is why I've created the *Man Diet*.

In this "diet" – and it isn't actually a diet, but a way of eating – you won't be limiting your calories, rather, eating certain macronutrients at certain times (unless you're carrying too much body fat).

You'll learn how to, as your ancestors did for eons, eat like a damn man!

You'll learn how to naturally enhance your testosterone levels, burn fat, build muscle, increase your energy, and bring your body back to where it should be.

If you're older, you'll feel younger.

If you're younger, you'll feel better.

If you're weak, you'll grow stronger.

If you're fat, you'll get ripped.

You'll hear this quote a few times over the manual,

but I use Abraham Lincoln to frame my view on nutrition when he said,

> *It's not the years in your life that*
> *count. It's the life in your years.*

In this diet we're going to show you how to *bring back your alpha*. We'll show you how to maximize your fat loss, by positively impacting your hormones, and not feeding your fat cells with highly glycemic carbohydrates, instead using these carbs at the right times to feed your muscles. We'll show you how to burn fat while building strong, athletic, alpha male muscle.

We'll provide you with the guidelines to create a way of eating, and a way of life that will improve your years, and add more of them, all wrapped in a way of eating that's sustainable.

One of the primary problems with most diets is that they aren't at all sustainable.

They recommend you restrict calories, which lowers your energy levels, raises cortisol levels, and makes you burn more muscle, while lowering your testosterone levels.

With *the Man Diet*, we're going to EAT LIKE MEN!

You'll eat your fill with every meal. You won't *over-eat* – because that's as destructive as under-eating. You'll do things "just right", and as you always *should have been* doing things.

The Diet That Isn't a Diet

While we're not going to restrict calories, we'll have guidelines to follow that will give you more freedom, but we're primarily simply going to eat the right calories at the right times.

Studies have shown that when you limit your caloric intake below what you're used to – by a wide margin – your body shuts down, stops burning fat, starts releasing cortisol, and intensifies whatever cravings for dirty, tasty foods that you may have already had.

There will be *no* calorie-restricting in the *Man Diet* to start (even if you're overweight, you're not going to *start* by restricting your calories). If your biggest barrier is that you're carrying too much body fat and it's increasing your estrogen levels, you'll reduce your caloric intake for a time, but the *kind* of calories you're going to be consuming, will, however, differ.

Forget about counting calories or measuring your food for now, you want to be at a caloric maintenance, especially before you start your caloric deficit if you're overweight. You need your metabolism to acclimate to eating the right macronutrients and the right amounts before you reduce anything.

The basis for our diet will come from our macros. You'll be consuming a diet based on the following macronutrient breakdown:

35-40% fats (varies depending on your goals)
25-30% proteins
35-40 % carbohydrates (cheat day not included, and varying depending on your goals)
(I use a 35(F), 35 (C), 30(P) breakdown)

Chapter 16
A Guide to Eating Like a Man

"Relieved of moral pretense and stripped of folk costumes, the raw masculinity that all men know in their gut has to do with being good at being a man within a small, embattled gang of men struggling to survive."

~ *Jack Donovan*

WE'RE GOING TO use an ever-more popular 'cheat' to ensure we're not eating too much, but instead almost blindly eating the right amount of food every day.

The cheat is called intermittent fasting, and while it's something I've used for the past few years, I'm not an expert on it. So, I teamed up with someone who is; Stephen Anton, Ph.D. Dr. Anton is a leading researcher on the benefits of intermittent fasting. Now, what he'll provide is invaluable to creating a routine that you can follow without much effort to achieve the optimal testosterone levels you need, crave, and damn well deserve.

Enter, Stephen Anton...

Ok, now it's time to talk about **Intermittent Fasting** and how it may be the missing piece to unlock your full potential as a man.

There are so many reasons to incorporate Intermittent Fasting into your lifestyle... if your goal is to create a healthy, strong, and powerful mind and body.

Before we get into the *Why and How of Intermittent Fasting*, we need to first dispel a few myths.

Myth #1. You need to eat every few hours or you will lose your precious muscle.

Contrary to "traditional" wisdom taught to bodybuilders over the past century, your body simply does not need to eat every three hours to maintain your precious muscle.

If this were the case, we would all wake up with less muscle than we had before going to bed. Of course, you know this does not happen. Rather, you are more likely to see your abs and also greater muscle definition upon rising in the morning. Not only that, but you probably feel alert, energized, and ready to take on the day... most days!

Why?

Well, when we sleep our bodies go through the very natural process of switching our energy source from glucose to fatty-acids and fatty-acid derived ketones (if you are a reasonably healthy man). Not only that, bodies repair and regenerate the vital tissues and organs, which occurs while we are fasting!

Most healthy men wake up in a state of mild ketosis. And that is a very good place to be from a fat loss and muscle gain perspective. We will discuss the amazing science behind this very natural process shortly.

Myth #2 – You should strive to be in an anabolic state all the time.

This one is laughable since you simply cannot be "anabolic" 24 hours per day. And spending some time in a "catabolic" state is critical to experiencing the full benefits of the anabolic time period. The key is to alternate one with the other and then watch your fat levels go down while your muscles grow… it's a beautiful thing.

In line with this, many top bodybuilders have said "Sleep is the most anabolic thing you can do for your body" – this may sound counterintuitive on the surface but in this section, we will explore the many reasons why good quality sleep combined with intermittent fasting represent the a potent anabolic combo (even though we recognize that these are technically "catabolic" activities).

In the sections below, we will go into detail about how critical the "catabolic" activities of sleep, fasting, and exercise (yes, exercise is a catabolic activity) are to your muscle growth.

Myth #3 – Breakfast is the most important meal of the day.

Most guys think that they need to eat very soon after awakening and/or the minute they feel a little hungry. By eating breakfast right away, they miss out on the many benefits that occurs from extending the fasting period to be 14-16 hours (or even longer) every day.

The key is to train your body to use your own fat and ketones, rather than your precious muscle, for energy. Then while you are fasting, your body goes to work repairing any muscle or tissue damage that occurred from your training sessions (see our recommended program), while simultaneously using your own stored fat for energy.

Not only that, but your body is in a similar state hormonally speaking as when you have just trained (low insulin but high growth hormone and testosterone levels). So you now have the potential to experience <u>two anabolic spikes</u> each day – one following your first meal after your 14-16 hours fast, and the other being your post-workout meal, if you train in the evening.

Does this sound too good to be true?

The good news is that it is not and scientific studies over the past century support the multiple benefits of Intermittent Fasting, particularly for men. Sometimes in life, the solutions are so simple that we miss them.

Let's get started

Ok, now that we have dispelled a few myths out there, we need to first define what we mean by Intermittent Fasting. You have likely noticed that lots of people are talking about "Intermittent Fasting" these days, but it can actually mean many different things.

The type of Intermittent Fasting we recommend would technically be called time restricted feeding. This essentially involves fasting for periods of approximately 16 hours and eating for approximately 8 hours EVERY DAY. We will discuss this approach in detail in the section below.

Another popular form of Intermittent Fasting is alternate day or alternate day modified fasting, which involves consuming no or very little food on fasting days and then alternating with a day of unrestricted food intake or a "feast" day. If your goal is strictly fat loss, then this option may be right for you. We summarize the science behind this approach at the end of this section.

If your goal is to lose body fat while preserving and/or growing new muscle, then read on to learn how this simple practice can transform your physique and also dramatically improve your health!

Remember earlier, we talked about the connection between body fat and your T levels (the more fat you have the lower your T levels). As we age, the connection between weight/fat gain, metabolic dysregulation and reduced testosterone become even clearer. In men between the ages of 40 – 79 years who were followed for about five years, researchers observed a direct connection between weight loss with a rise (and weight gain with a fall) in total T levels and Free T levels[A1] .

This is just one more reason why it is so important for you to lose body fat if you are currently more than 14% fat. By practicing Intermittent Fasting, your T levels will naturally go up due to the fat loss that will occur!

But why does Intermittent Fasting lead to fat loss and not muscle loss? The answer to this question is the focus of the section below.

We all naturally have the ability to train our body to use our own body fat for energy rather. And by practicing Intermittent Fasting regularly, your body can become more efficient at "flipping" this metabolic switch. When this switch is flipped, your body's energy source changes from glucose to free-fatty acids, **made from your own body fat**, and ketones, which serve to preserve muscle.

When your body's metabolic switch gets activated, the lipids in your adipocytes (fat cells) are then metabolized to free fatty acids, which are released into the blood. Simultaneously, other cell types may also begin generating ketones, with astrocytes in the brain being one notable example.

After reading this, you are likely wondering how you can activate your metabolic switch. Well, the good news is that this switch is likely turned on when you wake up every morning (or shortly thereafter), since this switch typically occurs after 8-12 hours of not eating.

We've briefly covered a number of benefits that an IF approach can bring, such as reduced glucose levels in the blood, increased insulin sensitivity (incredibly important in maintaining an efficient body), and increases in growth hormone levels that lead to both improved fat loss and reduced aging. But the benefits don't stop there...

Intermittent Fasting will improve *virtually every aspect of your health*! In the section below, we review some of the benefits that are not widely known.

First, Intermittent fasting helps your cells become healthier, which can reduce toxic load. During fasting, the process that your cells use to eliminate waste products, called ***autophagy***, is activated. This means you are cleaning out the "junk" when you are fasting, and this process appears to be critical to the survival of every cell in your body and has been linked to lifespan.

In fact, the Nobel prize was awarded to a researcher in 2016 for the discovery of autophagy and the connection between this cellular quality control process and virtually every aspect of our health.

What's more, **the process of autophagy is actually required to maintain muscle mass**. When autophagy was intentionally prevented in rodents, their muscles quickly atrophied and they became weak[A2] . This is actually not all that surprising when you think about it, since we know the importance of sleep to muscle growth, and for most people sleep is the time when autophagy is highest!

Findings such as this strongly suggest that any impairments in the cellular quality control system can accelerate the process of muscle degradation during aging! Not only that, but when this cellular quality control process is not functioning efficiently, your metabolism can actually slow down and set you up for unhealthy weight gain.

For most people living an unhealthy lifestyle, this process unfortunately declines with age, and leads to increased abdominal fat and muscle loss [A3]. Once accumulated, this excess body fat can further disrupt cellular quality control processes and set up a vicious cycle of fat gain and muscle loss [A4].

On the other hand, when you practice Intermittent Fasting, your cells can become healthier. And healthier functioning cells means that there are less "bad guys" around, which allows your body to use more of its resources to repair and recover instead of fighting the "bad guys."

Now, efficiency is something we've also talked about briefly thus far in the *Man Diet*, and an IF approach to eating will help your body eliminate waste that can also help speed up the healing and recovery process.

What's more, science has now revealed yet another amazing benefit of short-term or intermittent fasting, which is that it can dramatically increase the supply and availability of particular types of stem cells, called mesenchymal stem/progenitor cells, which decline during aging. (PMID: 26094889[A5]) In practical terms, this means that Intermittent Fasting helps your tissues repair and recover by increasing the supply and availability of stem cells.

In addition to the great benefits described above that occur at the cellular level, Intermittent Fasting has been shown to have broad systemic effects and trigger important biological pathways that promote health and optimize function.

Intermittent fasting regimens have consistently been found to decrease fasting glucose levels and reduce insulin resistance, as well as reduce both systolic and diastolic blood pressure and improve blood cholesterol levels. You may have heard of Insulin Resistance and how it can lead to type 2 diabetes. Well, the opposite of insulin resistance is insulin sensitive cells, and when you practice intermittent fasting regularly your cells become more insulin sensitive!

During intermittent fasting, plasma glucose, insulin, and leptin levels all go down, and ketone and adiponectin (fat burning hormone) levels go up, reflecting the body's switch in fuel source from glucose to fatty acids and fatty acid derived ketones. In a recent study, serum ketone bodies were almost 4 times higher when individuals followed a fasting mimicking diet compared to their normal intake. (PMID: 26094889[A6])

During fasting, growth hormone go way up [A7]. And we know that increased growth hormone levels change energy substrate utilization by liberating free fatty acids, and using these for energy in preference of protein. In order words, the increase in growth hormone during fasting increases lipolysis (fat burning) and also helps preserve your lean muscle tissue. This is likely one of the key mechanisms through which Intermittent Fasting improves body composition, which we discuss in more detail shortly.

Fasting also increases your body's glucagon. Glucagon is one of the dominant hormones in your body that's responsible for burning fat. This gives you one more tool that will help you burn fat, positively affecting your testosterone levels at the same time. Not only that, glucagon is a critical hormone for increasing satiety (feeling full), which may be one reason that many people do not experience hunger when they fast for short time periods (14-16 hours).

This all sounds great, but is there any scientific evidence that Intermittent Fasting can work for men who lift weights?

The answer is a resounding YES!

The findings of a clinical trial specifically conducted in men who practiced Intermittent Fasting and Weight Lifting are now available! In this study, 34 healthy men were randomly assigned to either a normal control diet or daily Intermittent Fasting (16 hours of daily fasting) and followed for two months during which they maintained a standard resistance training program, **the men in the Intermittent Fasting Group showed a reduction in fat mass (compared to normal diet) but no loss of lean mass or maximal strength.(125)**

Based on these findings, the scientists concluded "Our results suggest that an intermittent fasting program in which all calories are consumed in an 8-h window each day, in conjunction with resistance training, could improve some health-related biomarkers, decrease fat mass, and maintain muscle mass in resistance-trained males."

As great as these findings are, we believe you can do even better and pack on high quality muscle by taking advantage of the **two anabolic windows** that occur when you practice intermittent fasting with strength training.

As we mentioned earlier, the **first anabolic window** occurs immediately following your 14-16 hour fast. During this time, your body has utilized its glucose/glycogen supply and is burning fat for energy, which sets you up for a large anabolic response to your first meal.

Ok, but what should I eat for my first meal? Here, we recommend eating a meal comprised mostly of healthy fats with some protein and a small amount of carbohydrates… if your goal is to maximize fat loss and gain lean muscle. This type of meal will not only prolong the fat burning period, but also provide your body with a healthy supply of energy along with the building blocks it needs to grow and/or maintain muscle.

If you are less concerned about body fat, then you can be more liberal with the carbohydrate intake at this meal. The pro is that an increase in carbohydrate intake at this time could amplify the anabolic response by stimulating the hormone insulin and thereby potentially increase muscle growth. On the other hand, too many carbohydrates at this time can take you out of the fat burning state and trigger a metabolic switch for fat storage. It all depends on your goals!

The **second anabolic window** happens during the post-workout time period at night, presuming you train in the afternoon and/or early evening. After this workout, you get a huge insulin response at the time when your muscles are primed to absorb glucose to repair and regrow. So, during this post-workout anabolic window, almost all the glucose from carbohydrates is used by your muscles and does not stay in your bloodstream for long.

You now have "free reign" on your post workout meals. That is, eat however many carbs and proteins as you want.

Keep your fats low, but pig out on your post workout meals. Keep the rest of your meals big, but high in fats and low in carbs. This will likely lead to a break in your macros, which, to be honest, is fine. If you're going above and beyond with your carbs and protein in your post-workout meal, and your goal is to gain muscle, you'll be fine.

If your preference is to train in the morning, all is not lost. While you will not have two anabolic windows, your **post-training anabolic window** will be HUGE! That is, if you have fasted and/or had only amino acids before your morning training session. If so, then the next meal you eat will be critical to your muscle building success and should primarily consist of liberal quantities of carbohydrates (both simple and complex) as well as some lean protein.

A Bit More Science

In order to gain a better understanding of the effects of Intermittent Fasting on changes in body composition, Dr. Anton and his research team completed a systematic review of findings of clinical trials that were conducted in the past few decades. (Anton et al. XY) This article entitled *Flipping the Metabolic Switch: Understanding and Applying the Health Benefits of Fasting* was most downloaded paper in 2017 from the journal *Obesity* and can be found here[A8] - https://www.ncbi.nlm.nih.gov/pubmed/29086496

In addition to the Moro study (described above), three of four eligible trials showed that the Intermittent Fasting approach recommended in The Man Diet significantly reduced body weight and body fat in both normal weight and overweight men (and women). Importantly, no significant reductions in lean mass were reported in any study, which suggests the <u>weight losses were primarily comprised of body fat</u>.

Equally important, **the participants were <u>NOT</u> restricting calories during their eating window**. Earlier we discussed how restricting your calorie intake can LOWER your T levels. The good news is that by consistently practicing Intermittent Fasting, you get the fat loss benefits of calorie restriction, without the downside of LOWER T levels, as well as less lean mass, neither of which is good!

For studies involving Alternate Day Modified Fasting or Alternate Day Fasting, significant reductions in body weight and fat mass were observed in 10 of the 10 eligible trials. Yes, you read that correctly, 10 of 10 trials showed significant reductions in body fat. Additionally, the magnitude of weight losses were quite large with almost all of these trials reporting substantial reductions in body weight (> 10 lbs).

If you are a more visual person, the figure below summarizes the changes in body fat and lean mass that occurred follow studies using TRF and ADMF from Dr. Anton's review.

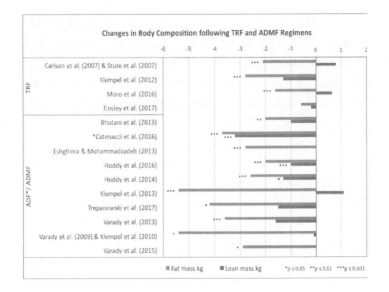

Changes in Body Composition following TRF and ADMF Regimens

So what does all this science mean for you?

Well, it means that a few things: 1) you have choices in the approach you take to Intermittent fasting, and 2) the type of program you choose should be based on both your goals and lifestyle preference.

The type of Intermittent Fasting approach we recommend of fasting for a window of 14-16 hours daily can clearly stimulate fat loss. And it can, actually be a great way to build muscle without gaining a bunch of fat like you'll see in bulking approaches that actually have a negative effect on the muscle-building hormone, testosterone. Additionally, it can produce amplify the release of growth hormone, which is known to have favorable effects on body composition.

If your focus right now is strictly fat loss, however, and

are as not as concerned about losing lean muscle, then the Alternate Day Modified Fasting approach would likely be your best strategy. With this approach, you would eat a very small meal (500 calories or less) during the afternoon one day, and then "feast" the next day. The good news is that as long you first completed the "fast" day, you can go wild on the "feast" day and eat until your heart is content. <u>The research is clear – you will indeed lose fat and relatively little muscle following this approach</u>.

It is, however, important that you do eat the small meal on your "fast" day. In the only study to look at the effects of Alternate Day Fasting (no calories at all on Fasting Days), the participants lost a significant amount of lean tissue (aka muscle)!

How to Adapt to Fasting Like a Man!

If you have read this far, we know that you are serious about incorporating intermittent fasting into your lifestyle AND are very committed to your own health. We are also committed to you becoming the very best version of yourself possible.

Even for a highly committed and health conscious individual, such as yourself, incorporating IF into your lifestyle will likely not be easy… at first. It can be a difficult transition from consuming five to six meals that are spread out over an entire day, then trying to nestle into an IF approach. As such. we have provided a list of strategies below to help you incorporate IF into your lifestyle.

But first, we think it is very important to have a short discussion on **perfectionism**. Perfectionism here will undermine your progress and wipe out long-term results. For this reason, we highly recommend NOT trying to be perfect with IF right from the start. The key is to come up with an approach that is sustainable…for YOU!

There are tremendous benefits to be had from simply doing IF every other day at first or gradually extending the time of your fast or having some cream with your coffee while fasting. Whatever it is for you, we highly recommend you do this during the adaptation period. Why? Because too many men and women fall into the trap of perfectionism and then abandon any positive lifestyle changes they made because they weren't "perfect."

This trap had ruined the otherwise successful path for an untold number of individuals and we do not want you to be one of them!

Ok, without further ado, here are a few strategies that can help you adapt, and eventually thrive using intermittent fasting:

Drink coffee. It's a natural appetite suppressant that will help you in your fasting phase. Not only that, there is now evidence that coffee can help your body produce ketones!

So it can help you get into ketosis and burn fat while preserving muscle.

Drink a ton of water. Drink at least 3 to 4 liters of water a day.

Ease into it. You don't have to dive right into the 16/8 model we're going to use. You can begin by simply delaying your breakfast, having it later and later in the day.

Stay busy. If you're not thinking about eating at the beginning of the day, you won't crave food. Make sure you stay busy to start your day.

Try it for at least 3 weeks. If you still can't get used to IF, and you need more frequent meals, then switch back, but make sure you give it 3 weeks.

Eat Green and Stay Lean. Before abandoning the plan completely, consider having some dark green vegetables or vegetable juice during the fasting period. Green vegetables have a very small metabolic effect and can help you feel full and energized during the fasting period. Of course, this would not technically be fasting but would be next best thing.

A Note about Your Food Choices. Just because you're IF, doesn't mean that you can eat crap. Sure, we're consuming a lot of great tasting food, but we're still trying to be healthier, stronger men. Eat clean. Live clean.

So... what is it that will make IF sustainable for you? *Will it require a change in lifestyle*? YES

Will it be easy? Probably not at first, but over time it will feel natural and leave you wondering how you lived any other way.

Will it be worth the effort? ABSOLUTELY

PART II

Implementation

CHAPTER 17
WHAT TO DO. WHAT TO AVOID. HOW TO EAT LIKE A MAN.

THE MAN DIET is split into two parts. The first aspect covers structure, the 'why', and what testosterone is, and how it affects your mind, body, and life. The second part is the boring but necessary aspect of what to actually eat, what to avoid, and how much to eat.

This section is filled with studies and lists of what to avoid and what to consume more of. It will simplify what you eat. It will answer whatever questions you may have about the myths out there as to what helps produce more testosterone and what diminishes it.

When you're eating like a man, you're eating a simple diet devoid of the crap that increases estrogen. It's simple. And this section will draw the battle lines between what you should eat and what you should avoid.

Let's get into it.

Foods that Boost Testosterone

The importance of fat in your diet to produce testosterone cannot be understated. This doesn't mean you're going to consume *every kind of fat*, however, and it also doesn't mean you're going to consume an *extreme* amount of fat.

In the Man Diet I prescribe a diet that's hovering around 35% of your calories from dietary fats. That's based off of a number of studies. The first study found that diets with under 20% of the calories coming from fats saw lowered testosterone levels than those with 40% fats.[1] Another study by Volek et al. again found the importance of dietary fats for testosterone, but also interestingly found – along with other studies – that a high protein to carbs - or - protein: fats ratio would create lower testosterone levels during rest than diets higher in carbs and fats, meaning that you're going to consume more carbs and fats than proteins.[2]

Step 1: Know Your Fats

First, after reading the first section of the Man Diet you'll know the importance of fats and of cholesterol. Where you get your fats and the foods you eat are, however, as important as the fat itself.

Take the vegetarian or vegan diet as an example.

You can consume fats from avocados and through supplementation, but you're not going to create as much free T or overall testosterone if you're consuming a healthy diet filled with vegetables and fruits *and meats*.[3]

Two other studies by Wang et al and Dorgan et al found a similar correlation between men who were given low fat diets versus men who were given high fat diets. Both found that the men who were on high fat diets had 12-13% higher testosterone levels, and higher free testosterone levels as low fat diets – vegan and vegetarian diets included – tend to produce more SHBG, a protein that bings to testosterone rendering it effectively useless to do what testosterone does. [4],[5]

There are also different *kinds* of fats, and not every kind of fat is good for you. In the list of foods that are testosterone-boosting vs the foods that are estrogen-boosting, you're going to see a solid grouping of fats.

If, however, you're consuming a nut or a food that you're not sure about, simply Google the nutritional facts for that food and see *which fats* it's predominantly made of. You'll see which ones to consume and which to avoid next.

Of course, as you're going to read, this doesn't mean that you have to freak out and only eat the fats that increase testosterone. All fats (except trans fats) are *good for you*. There are two that are better for your testosterone levels, but the third - as you'll read - is still an important part of your diet, you just don't need to dominate your diet with this form of fat like you're told to by some nutritionists and 'gurus'.

Testosterone-Boosting Fatty Acids

Saturated (SFA)

They're hard in room temperature (like when your bacon fat solidifies after being left on a cool pan). They're great for your testosterone levels and should be a healthy part of your diet. Animal fats are the best source, along with butter, dairy products, and coconut oil.

Monounsaturated (MUFA)

These are also great for your T levels and should be a healthy part of your dietary breakdown. They're liquid in room temperature, and include avocado and olive oil. Don't confuse these with PUFAs, which *are not* good for your T levels, and we'll talk about them next.

Another important note about MUFAs is their connection with vitamin E, which is an important one as shown by this study[6] that found that rats that were given vitamin E had significantly higher testosterone levels. It makes sense. Vitamin E is destroys harmful free radicals that would bind to free testosterone.

We're going to be talking about nutrients and foods that you can consume coming up, and you're not actually going to see vitamin E on the list. That's because, so long as you're getting your MUFAs, you won't need to supplement with vitamin E.

Testosterone-Killing Fats

Polyunsaturated (PUFA)

These too are liquid at room temperature, but they're not good for your T levels. They include canola oil, sunflower seed oil, fish, and margarine.

The reason for PUFAs not being great for testosterone is the fact that they're prone to damage when they get in contact with light, heat, or oxygen, the two latter being prevalent in the human body. When they come into contact with either of the above, they break down into harmful free radicals.

Important: I have also found a study that went against the consensus with PUFAs increasing T – though there's more evidence to suggest otherwise. With that said, I don't limit my fish intake. I take fish oil tablets daily because of their positive effects on brain health. You can go the extreme route and limit these fats from your diet, but a big part of our evolution as humans took place when we began to consume more fish. Just a thought.

Trans Fats

Of the fats mentioned, trans fats are the worst; they're also unnatural. Anything deep fried contains a hefty amount of trans fats and the foods you'll find in the freezer isles in your local market do as well.

More on Fats

One study found increased SFAs and MUFAs result in increased T production, but an increase in PUFAs resulted in suppressed testosterone production. [7]

Another study found placed their subjects on a diet where 40% of their calories were dietary fats, primarily from animal sources. They cut that amount to a low-fat diet where only 20% of their calories came from fat, saw the subjects testosterone levels plummet, then rise again once they were placed back on the 40% calories coming from fats diet.[8]

In short, consume a fair amount of SFA and MUFA fatty-acids while a moderate amount of PUFAs and no trans fats.

Step 2: Know Your Carbs

We've talked at length about fats because of their direct connection to producing testosterone. However, carbs are just as important because of their very direct relationship to cortisol.

Cortisol and testosterone oppose one another. Carbs help lower cortisol and help free you up to produce optimal testosterone levels.

For this reason, we're not going low carb. A study out of the University of North Carolina found that a low carb diet increased cortisol levels and decreased free testosterone levels.[9] Both Anderson et al and Volek et al found similar results in sedentary and resistance-trained subjects respectively, that both saw a decrease in free testosterone and and increase in cortisol with a low carb diet.

Just like dietary fats, not all carbs are good.

There's debate on this topic, but it makes sense that carbs that are higher in gluten and increase prolactin levels[10] (prolactin has a testosterone lowering effect[11]) would have a negative effect on your testosterone levels as well.

Things like grains and breads are also typically highly processed. It makes sense to follow a diet that primarily consists of things you can pick, pluck, or kill. A diet high in animals, fruits, veggies, and even things like potatoes, is ideal.

Don't, however, decrease your carb intake, following a primal diet that's devoid of carbs. Plenty of research is coming out showing that while animals are the most nutrient and calorically dense forms of food our ancestors had access to, they still ate plenty of fruits, veggies, and other sources of carbohydrates.

The aim for carbs is to be at about the 35% mark, along with your fats intake.

Here's the thing, we're all different. You may thrive off of higher fat and lower carbs or higher carbs and lower fats with higher protein (while studies suggest otherwise, there have also been compelling arguments for higher protein intakes and hormonal health because of the effects on body composition).

I like a balanced diet with a pretty balanced spread of macronutrients. If you're overweight, the first thing to do is to focus on getting your body fat percentage around the 10% mark so your caloric make-up will change. Carbs, no matter your goal, should be a solid part of your diet.

Chapter 18
How Much Should You Eat?

Since we're using an intermittent fasting (IF) protocol, meaning you're going to have a fasting and a feeding window, it helps to know just how many calories you need to be consuming. For a full list of resources, head to themandietbook.com/resources.

There you're going to find a few things.

1. You'll find a calculator that will help you determine how many calories you're burning in the run of a day (including activity and feeding).

2. You'll find a resource that will help you find, quickly, how many calories are in whatever food you're consuming.

IF is a powerful tool that helps guys burn fat without focusing too much on food intake. Being a fella who drinks a fair amount of coffee (which is an appetite suppressant), and who works a ton, I can go an entire day and forget to eat because I'm so into what I'm doing with my work. My issue isn't in calorie reduction, or having to reduce the amount of calories I'm consuming, but in eating *enough*.

Finding out how many calories I burn in the run of a day using a TDEE calculator, then doing a little bit of math to see if I'm hitting my mark, helps a lot. By now I have a good grasp on how much food I need to be consuming. But once or twice a month I'll run my daily meals through a calculator to figure out if I'm getting enough food in.

So what if you're overweight and you need to cut fat fast.

The first thing you're going to do is get your caloric intake up to a maintenance level. That is, you're going to eat the foods that boost testosterone, change the times you eat, follow the intermittent fasting protocol we've laid out, and allow your metabolism to once again regain its health and to run smoothly.

After you've been at a maintenance for 2 weeks, cut your caloric intake by up to 20% (start with 10%, then work your way up to 20%). You may not need to do this. With the increased activity levels and the IF protocol, fat loss may occur, we're going to hyperdrive fat loss to get you under that 14% body fat mark as fast as possible, then get back up to a caloric maintenance. These caloric deficits will be brief, so as to minimize the hormonal damage that can occur by dieting for too long. If you're dieting for too long, your metabolism is going to break down and you're going to have trouble losing fat as well.

Guys Who Need to Lose Fat

Since body fat is such a massive enemy of testosterone as it increases estrogen levels, there will be a large portion of guys who will have to cut fat before they settle into eating at a maintenance level for the remainder of their lives.

Keep this in mind, if you're not active, if you're not in the gym, you're not going to have optimal testosterone levels. Being active is a necessity. You need muscle. You need to be in shape. And being active is a necessary aspect of the Man Diet. With that said, assuming you're active and you just need to cut fat, we're going to do things a *little* differently (you can do the alternate day fast, or the following):

a.   *You're going to increase your protein intake and decrease your fat and carb intake. So you're going to have 40% of your calories coming from protein, with 30 coming from carbs and fats.*

b.   *You're going to start at the caloric maintenance (eating as much as you burn, which youll find out using the resources pages), but then you're going to cut calories so you can cut fat.*

While overeating is the more common mistake when cutting, some people tend to undereat. If taken too far, this can be worse than overeating because it can cause significant muscle loss. During your first week or two of cutting, you can expect to be a little hungry at times and to run into some cravings.

This doesn't mean that you're losing muscle or that anything else is wrong. It just comes with the territory, but it passes after a few weeks. A proper 'cut' is not supposed to be a grueling test of your will. When I'm cutting, I try to be within 50 calories of my daily target. Some days I'm a little higher and some a little lower, but I don't have any major swings in my intake.

Stick to lean sources of protein, and you won't have trouble putting together a meal plan that works. If your protein sources contain too much fat, you're going to find it hard to keep your calories where they need to be with proper macronutrient ratios.

After seven to ten days of sticking to your cutting diet, you should assess how it's going. Weight loss isn't the only criterion to consider when deciding if your diet is right or wrong, however. You should judge your progress based on the following criteria:

- *your weight (did it go down, go up, or stay the same?),*

- *your clothes (do they feel looser, tighter, or the same?),*

- *the mirror (do you look thinner, fatter, or the same?),*

- *your energy levels (do you feel energized, tired, or somewhere in between?),*

- *your strength (is it going up, going down, or staying about the same?), and*

- *your sleep (are you exhausted by the end of the night, do you have trouble winding down, or has nothing changed?).*

Let's talk about each point briefly.

If your weight is going up on a cut, you're eating too

much or moving too little. The exception, however, is when someone is new to weightlifting as he not only builds muscle while losing fat, which adds weight, but his muscles also suck up quite a bit of glycogen and water, which can easily add a few pounds in the first month.

Considering that you generally lose about 1 pound of fat per week, you can see how the fat loss can be obscured on the scale. So, if you're new to weightlifting and starting with a cut, I recommend tracking your waist measurement along with your weight for the first four to six weeks. If your waist is shrinking, you're losing fat, regardless of what the scale shows. In time, your muscles' glycogen and water levels will stabilize.

While you can continue building muscle while losing fat, you'll eventually lose more fat (in pounds) each week than you gain in muscle, resulting in net weight loss over time. If you're a more experienced weightlifter, however, and your weight is remaining the same after several weeks of cutting, you're likely just eating too much or moving too little.

Your waist measurement (at the navel) shrinking is a reliable sign that you're losing fat, so if your jeans are loosening, that's a reliable indicator of fat loss.

Your mirror, although it can be tough to observe changes in our bodies when we see them every day, you should definitely notice a visual difference after several weeks of cutting. You should look leaner and less puffy. If you don't, chances are your weight hasn't changed either or has gone up, and your jeans aren't feeling looser. This is a clear sign that something is off, and it's time to reassess your food intake or exercise schedule.

You should never feel starved and running on empty when cutting. Depending on how you ate before starting the cut, you may feel a little hungry for the first week or two, but after that, you should feel comfortable throughout the day. We all have high- and low-energy days, but if you're having more lows than usual, then chances are you're not eating enough or are relying on too many high-glycemic carbohydrates.

If you're new to weight training and start with cutting, you can expect to make strength gains. If you're an experienced weightlifter, however, it's normal to lose a few reps across the board when cutting, but you shouldn't be squatting 30 pounds less by the end of the first week. If your strength drops by a considerable amount, chances are, you're under-eating and need to increase your food intake.

If you're dead tired by bedtime, that's not necessarily a bad sign. It's common when people start training correctly. What's important, however, is that you sleep long and deeply. If your heart is beating quickly at night and you're anxious, tossing and turning in bed, and if you wake up more often at night, you might be overtraining or undereating.

Guys Who Want to Gain Muscle

Can you eat like a man and gain muscle? Of course. You obviously don't want to go crazy 'bulking', in fact, you may not want to 'bulk at all'. The reasoning is that testosterone helps you repair muscle tissue, and quite often - if you're not taking steroids - bulking (consuming a bunch more calories than you burn) can make you gain a bunch of fat, which will send your T levels plummeting.

The exception to this 'no bulking' rule are extremely skinny hardgainers. You're like I was. Every day I'd go to school with 7 sandwiches. I'd eat them all. Then I'd come home and polish off 3-4 servings of whatever my lovely mother had prepared for dinner. And yet, I couldn't get above 150 pounds.

If you're insanely skinny and you can't gain muscle, and you *want to gain muscle*, then eat like it's your job. Simple. Eat. Use the framework of the Man Diet but don't put a limit on your caloric intake. For the rest of you (us), myself included, eat at a caloric maintenance, but don't fret about going a tad over. The IF protocol and the macronutrients and the quality of the calories you're consuming are going to keep you lean.

The Rest

The Man Diet is really designed to be a maintenance diet. We're *using* IF to be able to eat more freely. We're consuming more of the foods that boost testosterone because things like animals taste delicious, and they're incredibly good for us.

Use the calculators that you'll find at themandietbook. com and figure out what your maintenance level is. Just as a gauge. And then eat and enjoy eating.

CHAPTER 19
TESTOSTERONE-BOOSTING FOODS

THE FOLLOWING FOODS help directly boost your testosterone levels because they're high in nutrients that help boost testosterone. Beside each food I'll put the ingredient or nutrient that they're high in (some are high in more than one) so you know *why* they're great for your testosterone levels.

First, however, let's cover the nutrients that will propel your T levels to new heights.

Fats (we've already covered this)
Carbs (we've already covered this)

Zinc

Zinc blocks aromatase, which is a precursor to estrogen. It also increases testosterone levels directly[12]. You need at least 15mg of zinc daily, and mega dosing has been shown to be fine in recent studies. You want to get your zinc levels tested before supplementing, but have at it. I included zinc in the Barbarian Manhood Multiy (averagetoalphasupple-ments.com) because it's one of the most important nutrients you can have if you want to maintain healthy testosterone levels (many of the nutrients and minerals you'll read about are in Barbarian).

Selenium

Selenium is a nutrient that's been linked to improved sperm quality and testosterone levels.[13]

Boron

Boron was found to increase free T in rats[14] and human subjects saw a 29% increase in T levels.[15]

Resveratrol

Increases the protein sTAR in cells, which enhances the conversion of cholesterol into testosterone and blocks the conversion of testosterone to estrogen.[16],[17]

Vitamin A

Vitamin A is an essential nutrient. Without it you'd go blind and become infertile. It's also been linked with increased testosterone levels.[18],[19],[20]

Vitamin K2

In two Japanese studies done on rats, the subjects T levels rose 70% in the blood and 90% in the testes.[21],[22] K2 needs to be researched more, but it also needs to be a part of your diet. Though we get K2 from leafy veggies, it's also important to supplement with it.

Vitamin C

Vitamin C is interesting. It protects testosterone cells from oxidative damage[23], lowers cortisol levels, improves sperm count and quality[24], but it isn't shown to directly improve testosterone levels. The positives demand that we supplement and consume it, however.

B Complex

B vitamins are involved in the synthesis of hormones and enzymes. You'll find them in eggs, meat, and other testosterone boosting foods.

Vitamin D3

D3 has been shown to increase free testosterone levels. While many suggest supplementing with 4,000IU daily, some evidence suggests we need up to double that daily.[25]

Magnesium

Like D3, magnesium increases free testosterone. Free T is the only form of T that's able to flow freely around the body, which makes it the only form of testosterone that truly matters. While you're focusing on overall T production, also focus on freeing that T up with magnesium and D3.[26]

Iodine

Iodine is closely connected to your thyroid health. A lack of it has been shown to cause hypothyroidism which lowers metabolic rate and testosterone.[27]

Pre and Probiotics

Not a 'nutrient', but gut health is increasingly being shown to help improve testosterone levels in men, even converting cortisol into androgens in the gut.[28],[29]

Now we'll get to the nitty gritty and go through foods you should have in your diet, and some you should avoid. There will be no 'conclusion' to this list because I want you to be able to print out the pages without having a bunch of useless literature from someone who just wants to hear themselves.

Estrogen-killing Veggies

Cruciferous vegetables are high in phytochemicals that block estrogen production. Be sure to have a healthy amount of these veggies in your diet. You can include them in smoothies and get them from a **good greens supplement**.

Cruciferous vegetables include:

- *broccoli*
- *cauliflower*
- *cabbage*
- *Brussels sprouts*

- *bok choy*
- *kale*
- *collard greens*
- *turnips*
- *rutabagas*

Fruits, Veggies, and Other Plants and Fungi

- *Pomegranate (boosted T by 24%[30])*
- *Red grapes (wine, raisins included) resveratrol*
- *Potatoes of all kinds (doesn't contain gluten, good for lowering cortisol)*
- *Cream of wheat*
- *Parsley (increases free T[31])*
- *Ginger (17% increase in T[32])*
- *Raw cacao (filled with T boosting fats and antioxidants)*
- *White mushrooms (block aromatase, the precursor to estrogen[33])*
- *Avocado (71% make up of t-boosting MUFA)*
- *Blueberries*
- *Blackberries*
- *Acai Berries*
- *Coconut/Coconut butter/oil (SUFA, MUFA)*

- *Onions (phytochemicals, antioxidants, one study found 300% increase in T[34])*
- *Coffee*
- *Olive oil (MUFA)*
- *Chia Seeds (have these instead of estrogenic flax seeds)*
- *Oats (I said no grains, but oats are filled with steroidal saponins that boost T)*
- *Tumeric[35]*
- *Cirtus Fruits (rich in antioxidants, very anti-estrognic)*

NUTS

- *Brazil nuts (SUFA, selenium)*
- *Macadamian nuts (SUFA)*

Most nuts are high in PUFAs, so opt for the nuts above. Avoid walnuts, pistachios, almonds, and peanuts, and each have been found to increase SHBG, the proteins bound to testosterone.

Meat, Dairy, and Other Animal Products

- *Yogurt (pre and probiotics are increasingly being shown to help boost T levels[36])*
- *Blue cheese (SUFA, probiotics, K2)*
- *Butter (SUFA, K2 opt for grass fed if possible)*
- *Oysters (zinc, selenium, vitamin D, copper)*
- *Animals*

I put animals in there simply to note that they are a testosterone superfood. All animals. Of course, opt for grass fed when possible, or even better yet, HUNT (the MUFA content in a wild animal is far higher than a farmed and corn-fed animal) as the quality of the meat is far better than what you'll find in a slaughterhouse.

Included in 'animals' is:

- *Bacon (naturally smoked or plain cut)*
- *Boar bacon (what I consume)*
- *Eggs (MUFA, SUFA)*
- *Elk*
- *Beef (grass fed beef is great for T)*
- *Venison*
- *Moose*
- *Bear*
- *Ram*
- *Bison*
- *Buffalo*

Depending on where you live and what you can hunt, get as much variety as you can. Increased variety in diet has also been shown to improve absorption of nutrients.

Foods That Hurt Testosterone and Libido

The following foods are high in phytoestrogens that can increase your estrogen levels. Here's the thing about phytoestrogens, depending on the person and their chemical make-up, they can actually help you flush out chemical estrogens. I haven't seen a test that helps determine which it will do for you, so I cut out chemical estrogens, buying natural cleaning products and avoiding plastics, and avoid these foods (except beer).

- *Soy*
- *Flax*
- *Beer/booze*
- *Beans/legumes*
- *Liquorice*
- *Fibers*
- *Processed grains*
- *Mint*

Foods That Stop Erectile Dyscfunction

When it comes to libido, there are a few factors at play.

For one, we need to boost testosterone – which we've already covered. Second, there are ingredients that link directly to increased sex drive (like ginseng) that we need to include in our diet. Third, however, and this will dominate the following section, we need to have foods that increase our blood flow.

As we get older many men have a problem getting it

up because of a decrease in blood flow. The best ingredient you can consume for increased blood flow and nitric oxide output, is citrulline.

Arginine is great, but it's precursor, citrulline, is more reliable. Foods like watermelon will give you a healthy *pump* both in your Johnson and in your muscles before a workout.

Include the following foods in your diet. They're both healthy and will enhance your libido. Go this route before you try male enhancement pills.

Improve Blood Flow

- *Beets are a great nitric oxide enhancer*
- *Garlic + Vitamin C combo boosting nitric oxide by 200%+*
- *Citrus Fruits*
- *Leafy greens*
- *Pomegranate*
- *Blackberries*
- *Watermelon – it's filled with citrulline, a precursor to nitric oxide*

Combating ED

- *Ginseng – you can supplement with it. Two studies, one with 900mg 3x per day, the other with 1,000mg 3x per day found that ginseng helped men get erect even with clinically diagnosed ED.[37],[38]*

Chapter 20
Your Simplified Schedule

I covered your schedule earlier, but it helps to have a very simple breakdown of how to optimally live to increase testosterone. These two schedules will help clarify when you eat what you eat and maximize every calorie you consume, you'll also see that there's a checklist to run through every day.

AM Workout

Rise
Push Ups
Cocktails
Workout
Carbs + Protein Shake
Carbs + Protein Meal
Move/Stand
Fats + Veggies Meal

Move/Compete
Fats + Veggies Meal
Journal/Review/3 Appreciations
Sleep

PM Workout

Rise
Push Ups
Cocktails
Fats + Veggies Meal
Compete/Work/Move
Fats + Veggies Meal
Workout
Carbs + Protein Shake
Carbs + Protein Meal
Journal/Review/3 Appreciations
Sleep

<u>The Testosterone Checklist</u>

Workout
Non-workout activity (walking, hiking, yard work etc…)

- *Workout (4 times a week)*

- *Compete (improve, fight, hustle)*

- *Winning (write down a daily victory)*

- *SLEEP 8 hours*

- *Sex (not porn)*

- *Consume a healthy amount of fats (40% of caloric intake)*

- *Consume ample amounts of cholesterol (eggs, bacon)*

- *Eat carbs (35-40% of caloric intake)*

- *Drink coffee (4mg/kg daily – 4 espressos)*

- *Hydrate (3-4 litres)*

- *Sprint (3-5 times a week)*

- *Choose your produce wisely (eat a lot of fruits and veggies, avoid pesticides)*

For a great resource on what foods boost and what foods hurt testosterone levels, check out anabolicmen.com. For another wonderful resources about vitamins and supplements and which ones work, check out examine.com.

Don'ts

- **Don't restrict calories (unless you're first focusing on fat loss)**

- **Don't consume too much alcohol (1-2 times a week, whisky over beer)**

- **Skim or Raw Milk (avoid whole, 2% pasteurized milk)**

- **Avoid these foods:**
  - *Green Tea*
  - *Soy products*
  - *Mint, spearmint, peppermint*
  - *Licorice*
  - *Flaxseed products*

- ○ *Trans-Fats*
- ○ *Alcohol (I don't avoid this completely, obviously, but opt for whiskey as often as possible over beer)*
- ○ *High-PUFA vegetable oils*
- ○ *High-PUFA nuts*
- **Don't run for long periods**

A point to reiterate…

I run for long periods. I may have booze a few times a week. Focus on the big things that will yield the highest returns. Workout. Sleep for 8-10 hours. Compete, hustle. Eat fats and carbs when they should be consumed.

Get after it.

Conclusion

'No man is more unhappy than he who never faces adversity. For he is not permitted to prove himself'

- Seneca

I DON'T KNOW what brought you here, to pick up a book called *The Man Diet*. My guess is that you're not a satisfied individual. You want to improve and you're looking for various ways to do so. Or maybe you're feeling lethargic, weaker, softer, and more sedated and you want to feel like the unstoppable man you once were.

Whatever brought you to pick up this book, I'm glad you did, and hopefully I provided the tools for you to unleash what should never have been bottled up.

Maybe this book simply provides permission to both eat and act like a man. Maybe it's a guide that will simplify your life, and help you live a stronger, more energetic and virile existence.

I cannot, however, leave *our* improvement confined to the pages of this book.

Hopefully by now you've headed to the resources section - themandietbook.com/resources - and signed up to the Man Diet Tribe newsletter. Let's continue what we've started in these pages. If there's anything I can help with, email me at chad@chadhowsefitness.com, and I'll respond as soon as I can.

The Man Diet is a way of eating that changed my life.

I was lethargic, sedated, easing into mediocrity, and turning my hormonal health around was the start to turning my life around. I'm ecstatic that I can pass this information on.

Now enough reading, get after it.

God bless,
Chad Howse

About the Authors.

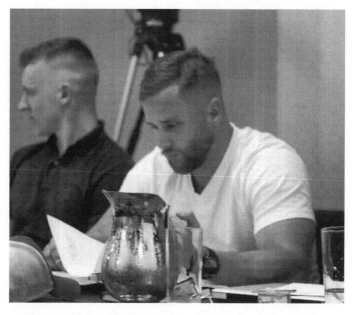

Chad Howse is the author of *the Man Diet*, creator of chadhowsefitness.com, average2apha.com, and Average to Alpha Supplements.

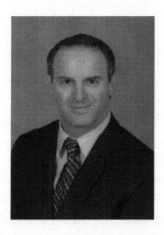

NAME: Stephen Anton TITLE: Associate Professor & Clinical Research Division Chief DEPARTMENT: Aging and Geriatric Research

BRIEF DESCRIPTION OF RESEARCH

Dr. Anton's specific research interests are in the role that lifestyle factors have in influencing obesity, cardiovascular disease, and metabolic disease conditions. He completed his doctoral degree in Clinical and Health Psychology at the University of Florida (UF), receiving training in health promotion and the delivery of lifestyle interventions designed to modify eating and exercise behaviors. Following completion of his post-doctoral fellowship at the Pennington Biomedical Research Center in June 2007, he accepted a joint Assistant Professor position within the Department of Aging and Geriatric Research and Department of Clinical and Health Psychology at the University of Florida. Since joining the University of Florida, he has successfully obtained and conducted multiple grants examining the effects that lifestyle-based interventions have on biological and functional outcomes relevant to obesity, cardiovascular disease, and metabolic disease conditions related to aging. With over 130 scientific articles and book chapters, his research has been recognized both nationally as well as internationally. In 2009, Dr. Anton was selected as an Outstanding Young Alumni by the College of Public Health and Health Professions. Then, in 2010, he was the recipient of the Thomas H. Maren Junior Investigator Award, which is awarded to one Assistant Professor in the College of Medicine each year. In 2013, he became the Vested Chief of the Clinical Research Division within the Department of Aging and Geriatric Research. During this same year, Dr. Anton was an Invited Member of the University of Florida's Leadership Academy. In June of 2014, Dr. Anton was promoted to Associate Professor with Tenure. In 2015, Dr. Anton was recognized as a Master Mentor by the University of Florida's Mentor Academy. Most recently, Dr. Anton was awarded a UF Term Professorship in 2017, a distinction given to top professors at the University of Florida.

Other books to read:

The Lost Art of Discipline by Chad Howse
Deep Work by Cal Newport
Essentialism by Greg McKeown
The One Thing by Gary Keller
Man's Search for Meaning by Viktor Frankl
How to Stop Worrying and Start Living by Dale Carnegie
Farther Than Any Man by Martin Dugard

Resources:

For research over the past decade I've used a TON of different resources. Here are the best ones:

www.examine.com

The 4-Hour Body by Tim Ferris

Man 2.0: Engineering the Alpha by John Romaniello and Adam Bornstein

www.ncbi.nlm.nih.gov/pubmed/

www.anabolicmen.com

www.poliquingroup.com

www.muscleforlife.com

CITATIONS

[1]Craig, B W, et al. "Effects of Progressive Resistance
Training on Growth Hormone and Testosterone
Levels in Young and Elderly Subjects."
Mechanisms of Ageing and Development., U.S.
National Library of Medicine, Aug. 1989, www.
ncbi.nlm.nih.gov/pubmed/2796409.

[2] Booth, A, et al. "Testosterone, and Winning and
Losing in Human Competition." *Hormones
and Behavior.*, U.S. National Library of
Medicine, Dec. 1989, www.ncbi.nlm.nih.gov/
pubmed/2606468.

[3] Coates J, Herbert J. Endogenous steroids and financial
risk taking on a London trading floor. *Proc Natl
Acad Sci U S A*. 2008;105(16):6167-6172.

[4] Bernhardt P, Dabbs J, Fielden J, Lutter C. Testosterone
changes during vicarious experiences of winning
and losing among fans at sporting events. *Physiol
Behav*. 1998;65(1):59-62.

[5] Booth A, Shelley G, Mazur A, Tharp G, Kittok R.

Testosterone, and winning and losing in human competition. *Horm Behav*. 1989;23(4):556-571.

[6] McCaul K, Gladue B, Joppa M. Winning, losing, mood, and testosterone. *Horm Behav*. 1992;26(4):486-504.

[7] Trumble B, Smith E, O'Connor K, Kaplan H, Gurven M. Successful hunting increases testosterone and cortisol in a subsistence population. *Proc Biol Sci*. 2013;281(1776):20132876.

[8] Salivary Testosterone Levels in Men at a U.S. Sex Club. SpringerLink. http://link.springer.com/article/10.1007/s10508-010-9711-3. Accessed February 4, 2017.

[9] Dabbs J, Mohammed S. Male and female salivary testosterone concentrations before and after sexual activity. *Physiol Behav*. 1992;52(1):195-197.

[10] Tsitouras P, Martin C, Harman S. Relationship of serum testosterone to sexual activity in healthy elderly men. *J Gerontol*. 1982;37(3):288-293.\

[11] Effect of cigarette smoking on levels of bioavailable testosterone in healthy men | Clinical Science. Clinical Science. http://www.clinsci.org/content/100/6/661. Accessed February 4, 2017.

[12] Smoking, sperm quality and testosterone level | Human Reproduction | Oxford Academic . Oxford Journals. http://humrep.oxfordjournals.org/content/17/12/3275.full. Accessed February 4, 2017.

[13] Testosterone and cortisol in relationship to dietary nutrients and resistance exercise. Journal of Applied Physiology. http://jap.physiology.org/content/82/1/49. Accessed February 4, 2017.

[14] Bélanger A, Locong A, Noel C, et al. Influence of diet on plasma steroids and sex hormone-binding globulin levels in adult men. *J Steroid Biochem.* 1989;32(6):829-833.

[15] Hill P, Wynder E. Effect of a vegetarian diet and dexamethasone on plasma prolactin, testosterone and dehydroepiandrosterone in men and women. *Cancer Lett.* 1979;7(5):273-282.

[16] DIETARY LIPIDS : AN ADDITIONAL REGULATOR OF PLASMA LEVELS OF SEX HORMONE BINDING GLOBULIN | The Journal of Clinical Endocrinology & Metabolism | Oxford Academic . JCEM. http://press.endocrine.org/doi/abs/10.1210/jcem-64-5-1083. Accessed February 4, 2017.

[17] Saturated fat and cardiovascular disease controversy – Wikipedia. Wikipedia. https://en.wikipedia.org/wiki/Saturated_fat_and_cardiovascular_disease_controversy. Accessed February 4, 2017.

[18] Dubois C, Armand M, Mekki N, et al. Effects of increasing amounts of dietary cholesterol on postprandial lipemia and lipoproteins in human subjects. *J Lipid Res.* 1994;35(11):1993-2007.

[19] Freedman D, O'Brien T, Flanders W, DeStefano

F, Barboriak J. Relation of serum testosterone levels to high density lipoprotein cholesterol and other characteristics in men. *Arterioscler Thromb*. 1991;11(2):307-315.

[20] Dietary Cholesterol Feeding Suppresses Human Cholesterol Synthesis Measured by Deuterium Incorporation and Urinary Mevalonic Acid Levels | Arteriosclerosis, Thrombosis, and Vascular Biology. ATVB Journal. http://atvb.ahajournals. org/content/16/10/1222.long. Accessed February 4, 2017.

[21] Testosterone and cortisol in relationship to dietary nutrients and resistance exercise. Journal of Applied Physiology. http://jap.physiology.org/content/82/1/49. Accessed February 4, 2017.

[22] Anderson K, Rosner W, Khan M, et al. Diet-hormone interactions: protein/carbohydrate ratio alters reciprocally the plasma levels of testosterone and cortisol and their respective binding globulins in man. *Life Sci*. 1987;40(18):1761-1768.

[23] Lane A, Duke J, Hackney A. Influence of dietary carbohydrate intake on the free testosterone: cortisol ratio responses to short-term intensive exercise training. *Eur J Appl Physiol*. 2010;108(6):1125-1131.

[24] Lee H, Ho C, Lin J. Theaflavin-3,3'-digallate and penta-O-galloyl-beta-D-glucose inhibit rat liver microsomal 5alpha-reductase activity and the expression of androgen receptor in

LNCaP prostate cancer cells. *Carcinogenesis.*
2004;25(7):1109-1118.

[25] Essayan D. Cyclic nucleotide phosphodiesterases. *J Allergy Clin Immunol.* 2001;108(5):671-680.

[26] Liao S, Lin J, Dang M, et al. Growth suppression of hamster flank organs by topical application of catechins, alizarin, curcumin, and myristoleic acid. *Arch Dermatol Res.* 2001;293(4):200-205.

[27] Human exposure assessment of fluoride from tea (Camellia sinensis L.): A UK based issue? ResearchGate. https://www.researchgate.net/publication/257422811_Human_exposure_assessment_of_fluoride_from_tea_Camellia_sinensis_L_A_UK_based_issue. Published May 1, 2013. Accessed February 4, 2017.

[28] McGregor S, Nicholas C, Lakomy H, Williams C. The influence of intermittent high-intensity shuttle running and fluid ingestion on the performance of a soccer skill. *J Sports Sci.* 1999;17(11):895-903.

[29] Liu T, Lin C, Huang C, Ivy J, Kuo C. Effect of acute DHEA administration on free testosterone in middle-aged and young men following high-intensity interval training. *Eur J Appl Physiol.* 2013;113(7):1783-1792.

[30] Hackney A, Hosick K, Myer A, Rubin D, Battaglini C. Testosterone responses to intensive interval

versus steady-state endurance exercise. *J Endocrinol Invest.* 2012;35(11):947-950.

[31] Nevill M, Holmyard D, Hall G, et al. Growth hormone responses to treadmill sprinting in sprint- and endurance-trained athletes. *Eur J Appl Physiol Occup Physiol.* 1996;72(5-6):460-467.

[32] Trunnelle K, Bennett D, Tulve N, et al. Urinary pyrethroid and chlorpyrifos metabolite concentrations in Northern California families and their relationship to indoor residential insecticide levels, part of the Study of Use of Products and Exposure Related Behavior (SUPERB). *Environ Sci Technol.* 2014;48(3):1931-1939.

[33] Larsen S, Spano M, Giwercman A, Bonde J. Semen quality and sex hormones among organic and traditional Danish farmers. ASCLEPIOS Study Group. *Occup Environ Med.* 1999;56(2):139-144.

[34] Allen N, Appleby P, Davey G, Key T. Hormones and diet: low insulin-like growth factor-I but normal bioavailable androgens in vegan men. *Br J Cancer.* 2000;83(1):95-97.

DIETARY LIPIDS : AN ADDITIONAL REGULATOR OF PLASMA LEVELS OF SEX HORMONE BINDING GLOBULIN | The Journal of Clinical Endocrinology & Metabolism | Oxford Academic . JCEM. http://press.endocrine.org/doi/abs/10.1210/jcem-64-5-1083. Accessed February 4, 2017.

[35] Bélanger A, Locong A, Noel C, et al. Influence of diet on plasma steroids and sex hormone-binding globulin levels in adult men. *J Steroid Biochem.* 1989;32(6):829-833.

[36] Hämäläinen E, Adlercreutz H, Puska P, Pietinen P. Decrease of serum total and free testosterone during a low-fat high-fibre diet. *J Steroid Biochem.* 1983;18(3):369-370.

[37] Cangemi R, Friedmann A, Holloszy J, Fontana L. Long-term effects of calorie restriction on serum sex hormone concentrations in men. *Aging Cell.* 2010;9(2):236-242.

Alcohol

[38] Välimäki M, Härkönen M, Eriksson C, Ylikahri R. Sex hormones and adrenocortical steroids in men acutely intoxicated with ethanol. *Alcohol.* 1984;1(1):89-93.

[39] Effects of acute alcohol intake on pituitary-gonadal hormones in normal human males. | Journal of Pharmacology and Experimental Therapeutics. JPET. http://jpet.aspetjournals.org/content/202/3/676.short. Accessed February 4, 2017.

[40] Sex hormones and adrenocortical steroids in men acutely intoxicated with ethanol. Alcohol Journal. http://www.alcoholjournal.org/article/0741-8329(84)90043-0/abstract. Accessed February 4, 2017.

[41] Effect of Moderate Alcohol Consumption on Plasma
     Dehydroepiandrosterone Sulfate, Testosterone,
     and Estradiol Levels in Middle-Aged Men and
     Postmenopausal Women: A Diet-Controlled
     Intervention Study. Online Library. http://
     onlinelibrary.wiley.com/doi/10.1097/01.
     ALC.0000125356.70824.81/abstract. Accessed
     February 4, 2017.

[42] Testosterone Increases in Men After a Low Dose of
     Alcohol. Online Library. http://onlinelibrary.
     wiley.com/doi/10.1111/j.1530-0277.2003.
     tb04405.x/abstract;jsessionid=B0E13DCD049
     737AC03BBE4DE9206648A.f01t01. Accessed
     February 4, 2017.

Jogging

[43] Wheeler G, Singh M, Pierce W, Epling W, Cumming
     D. Endurance training decreases serum testos-
     terone levels in men without change in lutein-
     izing hormone pulsatile release. *J Clin Endocrinol
     Metab*. 1991;72(2):422-425.

[44] Wheeler G, Wall S, Belcastro A, Cumming D.
     Reduced serum testosterone and prolac-
     tin levels in male distance runners. *JAMA*.
     1984;252(4):514-516.

Weight training

[45]Ahtiainen J, Pakarinen A, Kraemer W, Häkkinen K. Acute hormonal responses to heavy resistance exercise in strength athletes versus nonathletes. *Can J Appl Physiol.* 2004;29(5):527-543.

Intermittent Fasting

[A1] [A1]Camacho EM, Huhtaniemi IT, O'Neill TW et al. (2013)

Age-associated changes in hypothalamic-pituitary-testicular function in middle-aged and older men are modified by weight change and lifestyle factors: longitudinal results from the European Male Ageing Study. Eur J Endocrinol 2013; 168: 445-455

[A2]Masiero E, Agatea L, Mammucari C et al. Autophagy is required to maintain muscle mass. *Cell Metab* 2009;10:507-515.

[A3]**ingh R, Kaushik S, Wang Y et al. Autophagy regulates lipid metabolism. *Nature* 2009;458:1131-1135.**

[A4]**Verdejo HE, del CA, Troncoso R et al. Mitochondria, myocardial remodeling, and cardiovascular disease. *Curr Hypertens Rep* 2012;14:532-539.**

[A5]Cell Metab. 2015 Jul 7;22(1):86-99. doi: 10.1016/j. cmet.2015.05.012. Epub 2015 Jun 18.

A Periodic Diet that Mimics Fasting Promotes Multi-System Regeneration, Enhanced Cognitive Performance, and Healthspan.

Brandhorst S[1], Choi IY[1], Wei M[1], Cheng CW[1], Sedrakyan S[2], Navarrete G[1], Dubeau L[3], Yap LP[4], Park R[4], Vinciguerra M[5], Di Biase S[1], Mirzaei H[1], Mirisola MG[6], Childress P[7], Ji L[8], Groshen S[8], Penna F[9], Odetti P[10], Perin L[2], Conti PS[4], Ikeno Y[11], Kennedy BK[12], Cohen P[1], Morgan TE[1], Dorff TB[13], Longo VD[14].

[A6]

See 1 citation:

Cell Metab. 2015 Jul 7;22(1):86-99. doi: 10.1016/j.cmet.2015.05.012. Epub 2015 Jun 18.

A Periodic Diet that Mimics Fasting Promotes Multi-System Regeneration, Enhanced Cognitive Performance, and Healthspan.

Brandhorst S[1], Choi IY[1], Wei M[1], Cheng CW[1], Sedrakyan S[2], Navarrete G[1], Dubeau L[3], Yap LP[4], Park R[4], Vinciguerra M[5], Di Biase S[1], Mirzaei H[1], Mirisola MG[6], Childress P[7], Ji L[8], Groshen S[8], Penna F[9], Odetti P[10], Perin L[2], Conti PS[4], Ikeno Y[11], Kennedy BK[12], Cohen P[1], Morgan TE[1], Dorff TB[13], Longo VD[14]

[A7]M.L. Hartman, J.D. Veldhuis, M.L. Johnson, M.M. Le, K.G.M.M. Alberti, E. Samojlik, M.O. Thorner, Augmented growth hormone (GH) secretory burst frequency and amplitude mediate enhanced GH secretion during a two-day fast in normal men, J. Clin. Endocrinol. Metab. 74 (1992) 757–765

[A8]Obesity (Silver Spring). 2017 Oct 31. doi: 10.1002/oby.22065. [Epub ahead of print]

Flipping the Metabolic Switch: Understanding and Applying the Health Benefits of Fasting.

Anton SD[1,2], Moehl K[3], Donahoo WT[4], Marosi K[3], Lee SA[1,2], Mainous AG 3rd[5,6], Leeuwenburgh C[1,2], Mattson MP[3,7]

PART II CITATIONS

Diet

[1] Hämäläinen, E, et al. "Diet and Serum Sex Hormones in Healthy Men." *Journal of Steroid Biochemistry.*, U.S. National Library of Medicine, Jan. 1984, www.ncbi.nlm.nih.gov/pubmed/6538617.

[2] Volek, JS et al. *Testosterone and cortisol in relationship to dietary nutrients and resistance exercise.* J Appl Physiol. 1997; 82(1): 49-54

[3] Howie BBJ, Shultz TTD. Dietary and hormonal interrelationships among vegetarian Seventh-Day Adventists and nonvegetarian men. The American journal of clinical nutrition 1985;42:127-34.

[4] Wang, C et al. *Low-fat high-fiber diet decreased serum and urine androgens in men. J Clin Endocrinol Metab.* 2005; 90(5): 3550-9

[5] Dorgan, JF et al. *Effects of dietary fat and fiber on plasma and urine androgens and estrogens in men: a controlled feeding study. Am J Clin Nutr. 1996; 64(6): 850-5*

[6] https://www.ncbi.nlm.nih.gov/pubmed/6816576

[7] Volek J, Kramer W. Testosterone and cortisol in relationship to dietary nutrients and resistance exercise. Journal of Applied Physiology. http://jap.physiology.org/content/82/1/49. Accessed February 12, 2017.

[8] Hämäläinen E, Adlercreutz H, Puska P, Pietinen P. Diet and serum sex hormones in healthy men. *J Steroid Biochem*. 1984;20(1):459-464.

[9] [9] Lane, A R, et al. "Influence of Dietary Carbohydrate Intake on the Free Testosterone: Cortisol Ratio Responses to Short-Term Intensive Exercise Training." *European Journal of Applied Physiology*., U.S. National Library of Medicine, Apr. 2010, www.ncbi.nlm.nih.gov/pubmed/20091182.

[10] https://Fanciulli, G, et al. "Serum Prolactin Levels after Administration of the Alimentary Opioid Peptide Gluten Exorphin B4 in Male Rats." *Nutritional Neuroscience*., U.S. National Library of Medicine, Feb. 2004, www.ncbi.nlm.nih.gov/pubmed/15085559.

[11] Zeitlin, Scott I, and Jacob Rajfer. "Hyperprolactinemia and Erectile Dysfunction." *Reviews in Urology*, MedReviews, LLC, 2000, www.ncbi.nlm.nih.gov/pmc/articles/PMC1476085/.

Nutrients

[12] Kilic, M, et al. "The Effect of Exhaustion Exercise on Thyroid Hormones and Testosterone Levels of Elite Athletes Receiving Oral Zinc." *Neuro Endocrinology Letters.*, U.S. National Library of Medicine, www.ncbi.nlm.nih.gov/pubmed/16648789.

[13] Oluboyo, A O, et al. "Relationship between Serum Levels of Testosterone, Zinc and Selenium in Infertile Males Attending Fertility Clinic in Nnewi, South East Nigeria." *African Journal of Medicine and Medical Sciences.*, U.S. National Library of Medicine, Dec. 2012, www.ncbi.nlm.nih.gov/pubmed/23678636.

[14] "The Effect of Boron Supplementation on the Distribution of Boron in Selected Tissues and on Testosterone Synthesis in Rats." *The Journal of Nutritional Biochemistry*, Elsevier, 8 Dec. 1999, www.sciencedirect.com/science/article/pii/0955286396001027.

[15] http://www.bioimmersion.com/media/docs/fructoborate_monograph.pdf

[16] Wang, Y, et al. "The Red Wine Polyphenol Resveratrol Displays Bilevel Inhibition on Aromatase in Breast Cancer Cells." *Toxicological Sciences : an Official Journal of the Society of Toxicology.*, U.S. National Library of Medicine, July 2006, www.ncbi.nlm.nih.gov/pubmed/16611627.

[17] Wang, Y, and L K Leung. "Pharmacological Concentration of Resveratrol Suppresses Aromatase in JEG-3 Cells." *Toxicology Letters.*, U.S. National Library of Medicine, 28 Sept. 2007, www.ncbi.nlm.nih.gov/pubmed/17766065.

[18] Bishop, D T, et al. "The Effect of Nutritional Factors on Sex Hormone Levels in Male Twins." *Genetic Epidemiology.*, U.S. National Library of Medicine, www.ncbi.nlm.nih.gov/pubmed/3360302.

[19] Nayyar, T, et al. "Alterations in Binding Characteristics of Peripheral Benzodiazepine Receptors in Testes by Vitamin A Deficiency in Guinea Pigs." *Molecular and Cellular Biochemistry.*, U.S. National Library of Medicine, Aug. 2000, www.ncbi.nlm.nih.gov/pubmed/11055546.

[20] Zadik, Z., et al. "Vitamin A and Iron Supplementation Is as Efficient as Hormonal Therapy in Constitutionally Delayed Children." *Clinical Endocrinology*, Blackwell Science Ltd, 18 May 2004, onlinelibrary.wiley.com/ doi/10.1111/j.1365-2265.2004.02034.x/abstract.

[21] Ito, Asagi, et al. "Menaquinone-4 Enhances Testosterone Production in Rats and Testis-Derived Tumor Cells." *Lipids in Health and Disease, BioMed Central*, 13 Sept. 2011, www. lipidworld.com/content/10/1/158.

[22] "Vitamin K Deficiency Reduces Testosterone Production in the Testis through down-Regulation of the Cyp11a Cholesterol Side Chain Cleavage

Enzyme in Rats." *Biochimica Et Biophysica Acta (BBA)* - General Subjects, Elsevier, 6 June 2006, www.sciencedirect.com/science/article/pii/S0304416506001590.

[23] Vani, K, et al. "Clinical Relevance of Vitamin C among Lead-Exposed Infertile Men." *Genetic Testing and Molecular Biomarkers.*, U.S. National Library of Medicine, Sept. 2012, www.ncbi.nlm.nih.gov/pubmed/22731648.

[24] http://online.liebertpub.com/doi/abs/10.1089/jmf.2006.9.440

[25] Pilz, S, et al. "Effect of Vitamin D Supplementation on Testosterone Levels in Men." *Hormone and Metabolic Research = Hormon- Und Stoffwechselforschung = Hormones Et Metabolisme.*, U.S. National Library of Medicine, Mar. 2011, www.ncbi.nlm.nih.gov/pubmed/21154195.

[26] Cinar, V, et al. "Effects of Magnesium Supplementation on Testosterone Levels of Athletes and Sedentary Subjects at Rest and after Exhaustion." *Biological Trace Element Research.*, U.S. National Library of Medicine, Apr. 2011, www.ncbi.nlm.nih.gov/pubmed/20352370.

[27] Meikle, A W. "The Interrelationships between Thyroid Dysfunction and Hypogonadism in Men and Boys." *Thyroid : Official Journal of the American Thyroid Association.*, U.S. National Library of Medicine, www.ncbi.nlm.nih.gov/pubmed/15142373.

[28] Markle, Janet G. M., et al. "Sex Differences in the Gut Microbiome Drive Hormone-Dependent Regulation of Autoimmunity." *Science*, American Association for the Advancement of Science, 1 Mar. 2013, www.sciencemag.org/content/339/6123/1084.short.

[29] http://www.asbmb.org/asbmbtoday/asbmbtoday_article.aspx?id=48671

[30] Al-Dujaili, Emad, and Nacer Smail. "Endocrine Abstracts." *Pomegranate Juice Intake Enhances Salivary Testosterone Levels and Improves Mood and Well Being in Healthy Men and Women*, 1 Mar. 2012, www.endocrine-abstracts.org/ea/0028/ea0028p313.htm.

[31] Li, W, et al. "Effects of Apigenin on Steroidogenesis and Steroidogenic Acute Regulatory Gene Expression in Mouse Leydig Cells." *The Journal of Nutritional Biochemistry.*, U.S. National Library of Medicine, Mar. 2011, www.ncbi.nlm.nih.gov/pubmed/20537519.

[32] http://www.iasj.net/iasj?func=fulltext&aId=71548

[33] Grube, B J, et al. "White Button Mushroom Phytochemicals Inhibit Aromatase Activity and Breast Cancer Cell Proliferation." *The Journal of Nutrition.*, U.S. National Library of Medicine, Dec. 2001, www.ncbi.nlm.nih.gov/pubmed/11739882.

[34] Khaki, A, et al. "Evaluation of Androgenic Activity

of Allium Cepa on Spermatogenesis in the Rat." *Folia Morphologica.*, U.S. National Library of Medicine, Feb. 2009, www.ncbi.nlm.nih.gov/pubmed/19384830.

[35] Abarikwu, S O, et al. "Combined Administration of Curcumin and Gallic Acid Inhibits Gallic Acid-Induced Suppression of Steroidogenesis, Sperm Output, Antioxidant Defenses and Inflammatory Responsive Genes." *The Journal of Steroid Biochemistry and Molecular Biology.*, U.S. National Library of Medicine, Sept. 2014, www.ncbi.nlm.nih.gov/pubmed/24565563.

[36] Poutahidis, Theofilos, et al. "Probiotic Microbes Sustain Youthful Serum Testosterone Levels and Testicular Size in Aging Mice." *PLOS ONE*, Public Library of Science, journals.plos.org/plosone/article?id=10.1371%2Fjournal.pone.0084877.

[37] Hong, B, et al. "A Double-Blind Crossover Study Evaluating the Efficacy of Korean Red Ginseng in Patients with Erectile Dysfunction: a Preliminary Report." *The Journal of Urology.*, U.S. National Library of Medicine, Nov. 2002, www.ncbi.nlm.nih.gov/pubmed/12394711.

[38] de, E, et al. "Study of the Efficacy of Korean Red Ginseng in the Treatment of Erectile Dysfunction." *Asian Journal of Andrology.*, U.S. National Library of Medicine, Mar. 2007, www.ncbi.nlm.nih.gov/pubmed/16855773.